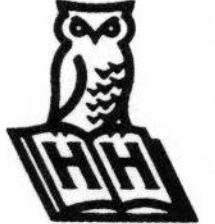

Say Good Night to Insomnia

Say Good Night to INSOMNIA

GREGG D. JACOBS, PH.D.

HENRY HOLT AND COMPANY NEW YORK

Henry Holt and Company, Inc.
Publishers since 1866
115 West 18th Street
New York, New York 10011

Henry Holt® is a registered trademark of
Henry Holt and Company, Inc.

Published in Canada by Fitzhenry & Whiteside Ltd.,
195 Allstate Parkway, Markham, Ontario L3R 4T8.

Library of Congress Cataloging-in-Publication Data
Jacobs, Gregg.
Say good night to insomnia / Gregg Jacobs.
p. cm.
Includes index.
ISBN 0-8050-5547-9 (hardcover : alk. paper)
1. Insomnia—Popular works. I. Title.
RC548.J33 1999
616.8'498—dc21 98-13112

Henry Holt books are available for special promotions
and premiums. For details contact: Director, Special Markets.

First Edition 1998

Designed by Paula Szafranski

Printed in the United States of America
All first editions are printed on acid-free paper. ∞

10 9 8 7 6 5 4 3 2 1

To my parents, for giving so much of themselves,
and to Jody, Lauren, and Andrew,
for making every day magical.

In memory of Richard Friedman,
whose brilliance, energy, and spirit
will live forever.

Contents

Foreword viii

Introduction Conquer Insomnia and Change Your Life x

Part I • Getting Started

Chapter 1. You *Can* Say Good Night to Insomnia 5

Chapter 2. Some Basic Facts About Sleep and Insomnia 14

Chapter 3. Putting Sleeping Pills to Rest 29

Chapter 4. Conducting Your Own Insomnia Self-Assessment 45

Part II • Changing Sleep Thoughts and Behaviors

Chapter 5. Changing Your Thoughts About Sleep 71

Chapter 6. Establishing Sleep-Promoting Habits 90

Chapter 7. Lifestyle and Environmental Factors That Affect Sleep 105

Part III • Managing Insomnia by Managing Stress

Chapter 8. The Relaxation Response 131

Chapter 9. Learning to Think Away Your Stress 156

Chapter 10. Developing Stress-Reducing, Sleep-Enhancing Attitudes and Beliefs 173

Appendix A. Managing Shift Work 193

Appendix B. Managing Jet Lag 197

Appendix C. Infants' and Children's Sleep 201

Appendix D. Additional Relaxation Scripts 207

Sources and Suggested Reading 212

Acknowledgments 217

Foreword

My first meeting with Dr. Gregg Jacobs was a memorable one. He had just completed his doctoral research—a groundbreaking study on the effects of the relaxation response on brain waves—and was applying for a postdoctoral fellowship under my direction at Harvard Medical School. I was so impressed with Dr. Jacobs that I not only offered him the fellowship but also invited him to accompany me and my research team on an expedition to India and Sikkim to perform physiological studies on the meditative practices of Tibetan monks.

Soon thereafter Dr. Jacobs began to investigate what would become a primary focus of his career: the nondrug treatment of insomnia using the relaxation response and other cognitive-behavioral techniques. He eventually developed the only nondrug treatment scientifically proven to teach insomniacs to become normal sleepers: 100 percent of patients treated with this intervention report improved sleep, 75 percent become normal sleepers, and 90 percent reduce or eliminate sleeping pills.

Using this treatment, Dr. Jacobs developed the Behavioral Medicine Insomnia Program at Harvard Medical School's Deaconess Hospital in Boston in 1991, the first nondrug insomnia program of its kind in the country. Since then, Dr. Jacobs has taught his insomnia program to thousands of individuals, including his patients, employees of major corporations, and health care practitioners. So successful is his insomnia treatment that the National Institutes of Health recently awarded him a prestigious four-year grant to compare the effectiveness of his treatment to sleeping medication. As Dr. Jacobs's mentor, I have taken pride in watching him distinguish himself as scientist and clinician.

With the publication of *Say Good Night to Insomnia*, individuals everywhere who suffer from insomnia can now benefit from Dr. Jacobs's program. In this book, Dr. Jacobs uses case examples and interactive exercises to clearly and concretely tell you what you need to do to conquer insomnia and how to do it. In a user-friendly, practical, organized fashion, he expertly guides you through a thorough six-week program for overcoming insomnia that parallels the program he developed here at the Harvard Medical School. You will also find that *Say Good Night to Insomnia* is more than just a book about insomnia; it is a book about improving yourself and your life. In it, you will learn scientifically proven relaxation response and stress reduction techniques for achieving greater mind-body control and improving your health and well-being.

Say Good Night to Insomnia reflects Dr. Jacobs's commitment and dedication to his patients as well as his experience, enthusiasm, and wisdom as a clinician and scientist. His program represents not only the future treatment of insomnia; it is the approach that should be adopted by all health care practitioners. Insomniacs everywhere finally have a safe, highly effective alternative to sleeping pills. I am confident that this program will change your life as it has for so many of Dr. Jacobs's patients.

—Herbert Benson, M.D.
Boston, Massachusetts
April 23, 1998

Introduction: Conquer Insomnia and Change Your Life

This book is about conquering insomnia. It is also about changing yourself and your life in more fundamental and powerful ways.

In our rapidly changing, stress-filled world, insomnia has become an epidemic. Half of all adults now complain of trouble sleeping, up from one-third just a few years ago. At least 30 million adults endure the stress of severe, chronic insomnia.

Yet despite the pervasiveness of insomnia in today's society, it has been largely ignored by the medical community. The National Institutes of Health have granted almost no funding for insomnia research, while medical schools teach virtually nothing about sleep or insomnia. The result, unfortunately, is that insomniacs have been left with two alternatives: take sleeping pills or live with the problem.

However, due to their potentially serious side effects and ineffectiveness with habitual use, it has become increasingly clear that sleeping pills are not the solution to insomnia. And, frankly, who wants to take sleeping pills for the rest of his or her life? We also know that it is possible to successfully treat insomnia with the step-by-step drug-free program described in this book; insomniacs, at last, can get the effective treatment they have long deserved.

Although there is an increasing number of articles and books about insomnia, few are based on the scientific research and clinical practice as that conducted by the author. This drug-free program is based on research and clinical practice that I have conducted over the past ten years at Harvard Medical School. It is the *only* drug-free program scientifically proven to help insomniacs become normal sleepers. Not only have 100 percent of the patients treated with this program reported improved sleep; 90 percent have also decreased or eliminated use of sleeping pills. And, unlike sleeping pills, which cannot claim these results, this program has no side effects except significantly improved sleep, mood, and energy; it is also safe, and less expensive and more effective than sleeping pills.

This book is not just about conquering insomnia. By learning to sleep well, you will also feel more energy and joy, and be more productive; feel calmer and more optimistic, and cope better; and enjoy being around others, who will then enjoy being around you—your relationships will improve.

The program will also teach you clinically and scientifically proven relaxation and stress-reduction techniques. These will improve your sleep and will help you:

- Handle negative emotions and stress-related symptoms more effectively, including headaches, gastrointestinal problems, anxiety, and anger
- Strengthen the functioning of your immune system and improve your health
- Quiet and control your mind and body and heighten peace of mind
- Think more positively and optimistically, which are traits now recognized as improving emotional well-being and physical health
- Realize the powerful effect your mind has on your emotions and health and that you possess the ability to alter and control events in your mind and body

By learning to successfully use the techniques in this program to take control of your sleep, mind, and body, you will be empowered by the realization that the key to conquering insomnia resides *within you*. Therefore, you will boost your confidence in your personal power and strengthen your sense of self-esteem, which is fundamental to optimal health and well-being.

In short, this book can be a catalyst for transforming yourself and your life on many levels.

As a clinician and scientist, I have enjoyed writing this book, for it has permitted me to write about a program that has transformed the lives of many of my insomnia patients and share it with many more sufferers. I am also excited because, even though many medical problems are now being treated effectively with behavioral medicine, or mind-body interventions, insomnia represents probably the most successful application of these techniques. This is why I believe insomnia is an exemplary model for understanding the connections between mind, body, and health.

I firmly believe in these techniques. You see, I, too, experienced a period of insomnia in my life and know firsthand the stress it can cause. By using these techniques, I overcame insomnia! I have also experienced the powerful impact these techniques can have, particularly those for relaxation and stress reduction, on the mind and body. For me, they represent an important component of a self-help approach to health and well-being.

How I Developed the Program

As an undergraduate psychology major, I took several academic courses on biofeedback and relaxation techniques. (I'll discuss these techniques in detail in chapter 8.) In one of these courses, I read about the pioneering work of Dr. Herbert Benson, whose research at Harvard Medical School on relaxation techniques was recognized internationally and described in his best-selling book *The Relaxation Response*.

I was fascinated by Dr. Benson's work, which was the first sound scientific research to demonstrate that it was possible to use the mind to modify the physiology of the body. At the same time, sensory isolation tanks, also known as flotation tanks, were being marketed as a new relaxation device. The idea underlying these tanks was straightforward: by floating on salt water in a quiet, dark, temperature-controlled environment, a deep state of relaxation could be attained. However, no one had ever conducted a controlled scientific study to ascertain whether these tanks were truly effective. I decided to conduct my own original research on relaxation techniques and to write an undergraduate senior honors thesis on the subject. Therefore, I built a sensory isolation tank and conducted the first scientific study on the physiological effects of the tank.

As part of this research, Dr. Alan Belden, the medical director of a stress-management clinic at a local hospital, allowed me to use his clinic's biofeedback equipment to measure the tank's physiological effects. I found that regular use of the tank produced reliable reductions in blood pressure and muscle tension in my subjects. As an undergraduate, I was fortunate to be able to publish my findings in the scientific journal *Health Psychology*.

I was a placekicker on my college football team and used the isolation tank myself to visualize and mentally rehearse my placekicking the night before football games. Two of my teammates, both running backs, also used the tank to mentally rehearse their running skills. By and large, this idea seemed to work: I became a record-setting all-conference placekicker, and my two teammates became all-Americans and received tryouts with professional football teams!

As it turned out, when I graduated Dr. Belden hired me to work in his clinic as a stress-management specialist and to set up the isolation tank. For the next four years, I worked closely with Dr. Belden using biofeedback, relaxation techniques, and the isolation tank to treat patients with various stress-related health conditions, including headaches, gastrointestinal problems, and anxiety.

This work presaged my later work with insomnia for important reasons: it provided me with convincing evidence that patients with stress-related health problems could use relaxation techniques to effectively manage those problems, and many of the patients told me they were able to use the techniques to become drowsy or fall asleep and sleep better at night.

I was so intrigued by these findings that, when I entered graduate school a few years later, I decided to conduct my doctoral dissertation on the effects of relaxation techniques on brain waves. In the study, which was one of the first of its kind and which would set the stage for my eventual research with insomnia, I discovered that college students were able to use relaxation techniques to voluntarily produce brain-wave patterns that were identical to the initial stages of sleep. I published my findings, which provided scientific proof that relaxation techniques produce measurable effects in the brain, in the journal *Behavioral Medicine*.

When I completed my doctoral dissertation, I wrote to Dr. Benson and described my research and my desire to work with him at Harvard Medical School as a postdoctoral fellow. After meeting with him, he not only offered me a fellowship, he also asked me to accompany him and a team of scientists on a research expedition to India and Sikkim to study the meditative practices of Tibetan monks who had previously been filmed engaged in an extraordinary meditative practice. In temperatures of 40 degrees Fahrenheit and dressed only in a loin cloth, each monk wrapped his body in a sheet soaked in ice water. Using their meditative powers, the monks then proceeded to raise their body temperature and steam the sheets dry! Because of the implications this had for understanding mind-body control and its application to Western medicine, we wanted to document the physiological changes associated with this meditative practice.

This was a memorable expedition. It not only afforded me the opportunity to visit India and the Himalayas, but I also had the privilege of meeting the Dalai Lama, the spiritual leader of Tibet. He facilitated the expedition and arranged for our team to spend several days at a monastery situated in the foothills of the Himalayas.

We measured the monks' ability to use meditative practices to control their physiological activity. My particular role in this research was to measure the monks' brain-wave changes. We found evidence that the monks could use their mental powers to voluntarily control their brain-wave patterns and oxygen consumption during meditation, which provided further scientific evidence that it was possible to use the mind to control the body. We published our findings in *Behavioral Medicine*.

In addition to my research fellowship with Dr. Benson, I was also awarded a postdoctoral clinical fellowship in the Behavioral Medicine Clinic at Children's Hospital of Harvard Medical School. This fellowship provided me the opportunity to use biofeedback and relaxation techniques to help children and adolescents manage a variety of stress-related medical symptoms including chronic pain, headaches, irritable bowel syndrome, colitis, and hypertension. As a result of this work, I became increasingly interested in the application of relaxation and mind-body techniques to clinical problems.

Around this time, I was contacted by Dr. Paul Rosenberg, a physician and specialist in sleep disorders at Harvard Medical School, who wondered whether I might be able to apply my research on relaxation techniques to help insomnia patients. I realized this was an excellent opportunity to work on a widespread health problem and decided to pursue this path as part of my postdoctoral research.

After reviewing all the existing scientific research on the use of relaxation and nondrug techniques for insomnia, two things became very evident. First, although relaxation and behavioral techniques had been used in the treatment of insomnia, no one had developed an effective nondrug intervention that allowed insomniacs to become normal sleepers; in other words, insomniacs in these studies slept better but still had insomnia. Second, insomnia is a learned health problem that is caused by thoughts and behaviors.

I became convinced that it was possible to develop a nondrug program that could actually help insomniacs become normal sleepers. Therefore, I developed the first drug-free intervention that incorporated relaxation and other nondrug techniques to treat the thoughts and behaviors that cause insomnia.

I then tested the effectiveness of this intervention by conducting a scientific study in collaboration with Dr. Rosenberg and other colleagues. Using sleep diaries, we found that insomnia patients who had previously required almost eighty minutes per night on average to fall asleep were able to do so in less than twenty minutes as a result of this drug-free treatment! This study, which I published in the journal *Behavior Modification*, demonstrated for the first time that it was possible to teach insomniacs to become normal sleepers using nondrug techniques.

Encouraged by these findings, I refined and improved these techniques, then conducted another scientific study in which I used brain-wave recordings to compare good sleepers to chronic insomniacs who were treated with this method. These insomniacs, who averaged one and a quarter hours per night to fall asleep and who had experienced insomnia for an average of eleven years, achieved the following remarkable results:

- They learned to fall asleep in less than twenty minutes and became indistinguishable from good sleepers
- Their sleep quality, mood, and daytime functioning also improved significantly and became equivalent to those of good sleepers
- They were more mentally relaxed in bed, as measured by slower brain waves
- Their improved sleep was maintained through long-term follow-ups

This study, which I published in the journal *Behavior Therapy*, again demonstrated that insomniacs could become normal sleepers using natural, safe, nondrug techniques.

When I completed my postdoctoral fellowship in 1989, Dr. Benson offered me a full-time appointment at Harvard Medical School as an Instructor in Medicine and a position in the Division of Behavioral Medicine at Deaconess Hospital. For the next seven years, I developed and directed the Behavioral Medicine Insomnia Program, which was based on my drug-free insomnia intervention. After successfully treating many patients in this program, I conducted a subsequent scientific study in which I documented that 100 percent of the patients—including those who couldn't fall asleep at bedtime and those who woke up during the night and couldn't fall back to sleep—reported improved sleep. Moreover, the majority of these patients reported at long-term follow-up that the improvements continued. These results, which I published in *The American Journal of Medicine*, were exceptional, considering that these patients had endured insomnia for an average of ten years and most had tried psychotherapy and sleeping pills without success before coming to my program.

I have now taught my program to thousands of individuals, including the insomnia patients I currently treat in the Sleep Disorders Center at the Beth Israel Deaconess Medical Center; health care professionals; and employees of major corporations such as Fidelity Investments, Reebok International, John Hancock Insurance Company, Texas Instruments, and Lotus Corporation. I have continued to refine and improve the program, finally arriving at the step-by-step self-help insomnia program presented here.

This book has been written to be practical and user-friendly. In it, I explain what you need to know about conquering insomnia without a lot of superfluous information. The book is organized in three parts:

Part I examines why medicine has failed insomniacs, and, in particular, why sleeping pills are not the solution. It also reviews research on this program, what it will do for you, and why it achieves its groundbreaking results. You will learn basic facts about sleep that are essential in understanding and using the techniques and in cultivating a sense of control over sleep. You will also learn how to perform your own insomnia self-assessment, which will help you identify the particular causes of your insomnia and ascertain whether medical or mental health problems may be contributing to it. I also review the various types of sleeping pills, their side effects, and, most notably, how to eliminate their use.

Part II explores sleep-promoting habits and health practices. You will learn to sleep better by modifying the way you think about sleep (cognitive restructuring), and learn to establish healthy sleep behaviors. How to use exercise, food, and light to improve sleep and how to minimize the detrimental effects of alcohol, caffeine, and nicotine will also be examined.

Part III explores the latest scientific research on stress and its effects on sleep. I will discuss three methods for reducing stress and enhancing mind-body control that will improve your sleep and health: the relaxation response, cognitive stress management techniques, and development of stress-resistant attitudes and beliefs.

Parts II and III consist of a total of six chapters that are designed to be implemented in a six-week program:

WEEK	CHAPTER	TOPIC
One	Five	Changing Your Thoughts About Sleep
Two	Six	Establishing Sleep-Promoting Habits
Three	Seven	Lifestyle and Environmental Factors That Affect Sleep
Four	Eight	The Relaxation Response

WEEK	CHAPTER	TOPIC
Five	Nine	Learning to Think Away Your Stress
Six	Ten	Developing Stress-Reducing, Sleep-Enhancing Attitudes and Beliefs

Although this book is for people who experience persistent problems falling asleep or who regularly wake during the night, it is also for those who wish to prevent occasional insomnia from becoming chronic and for those who simply want to sleep better. Part III can also be used by those who want to learn stress-reduction techniques for improved control over mind, body, and health.

This program is designed to be easy to learn. However, you must contribute by putting the program into practice. Like exercising, losing weight, or modifying other lifestyle behaviors, this program requires some effort and practice. Though it may not be as simple as taking a sleeping pill, the outcome—a good night's sleep, heightened mind-body control, and better health and well-being—make this one of the best time investments of your life.

To help you successfully use the program, I share case examples of patients who have utilized these techniques to master insomnia. Also included are interactive exercises, including a daily 60-Second Sleep Diary and a Weekly Progress Summary, that will enhance your understanding and use of these techniques.

In the appendices are relaxation scripts and helpful techniques for managing jet lag and shift work, and for improving sleep in infants and young children.

In as little as a few days, you will rediscover the pleasure of a good night's sleep. Within a few weeks, your mood and energy will improve. And, by the end of the program, you will look at yourself in a new and powerful way, and possess greater control over your emotions and health and greater control over life.

Say Good Night
to Insomnia

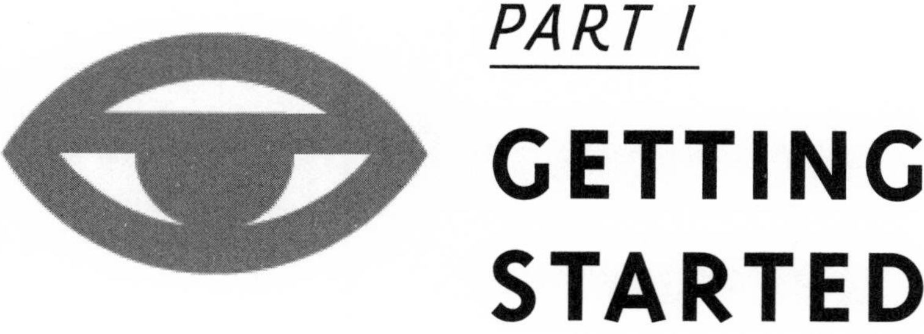

PART I

GETTING STARTED

CHAPTER ONE

You *Can* Say Good Night to Insomnia

Bedtime is approaching and Alan is dreading it. He knows what tonight will bring: the torment of another night of insomnia.

Each night has become agonizingly familiar. Exhausted, Alan gets into bed and turns out the lights to go to sleep, only to lie wide awake. The harder he tries to fall asleep, the more he tosses and turns and the more tense and frustrated he feels. With the realization that he can't fall asleep comes a distressing wave of anxiety and stressful thoughts about sleep—"I've got to get some sleep or I'll never function tomorrow!"—and the worries about the problems in his life: tomorrow's meeting, Friday's deadline, his company's downsizing, his mother's illness. All are made worse by the loneliness and darkness of the night.

Even when Alan finally falls asleep he cannot escape insomnia. After just a few hours, he wakes up and tosses and turns before falling back to sleep just as the sun rises.

When the alarm clock rings, Alan has to drag himself out of bed, angry and depressed in the knowledge that yet another day feeling wiped out, helpless, and desperate awaits him.

Insomnia has become Alan's living nightmare.

• • •

Does Alan's ordeal sound familiar? It does for most insomniacs, who live in an interminable state of anxiety concerning insomnia and its effects on their lives. Like Alan, they also feel hopeless, powerless, and trapped by their lack of control over sleep, and they dread what, for most people, is an enjoyable experience—going to bed.

And no wonder. The anger, exhaustion, and irritability caused by insomnia can handicap mood, productivity, coping skills, and family and social life, and deprive insomniacs of a sense of joy and well-being. They grow even more frustrated or depressed by family or friends who tell them "it's all in your head" or "just relax," and may start to wonder whether they have a "psychological" problem. As a consequence, insomniacs feel embarrassed or even ashamed about their condition, which diminishes their self-esteem.

Doctors and Sleeping Pills

It is stressful enough to endure insomnia, but many doctors' reactions to it can make it even worse. They frequently don't ask about insomnia, overlook it, or simply ignore it. Why? Because insomnia is so ubiquitous that it is often dismissed by doctors as an unavoidable and normal part of life!

Doctors are not trained to diagnose or treat insomnia. Even though it is one of the most frequent health complaints today, doctors receive less than one hour of training on sleep problems during their entire medical education. This lack of training is compounded by the fact that, until recently, little federal funding has been allocated for insomnia research, which means that information about treating insomnia is not available to doctors in medical and scientific journals. (Fortunately, Congress and the National Institutes of Health have started to appropriate more money for sleep and insomnia research, as evidenced by the recent decision to fund my own research for four years.)

It is easy to understand why doctors are not comfortable treating insomnia. And when they are not comfortable treating something, they are inclined to avoid it. As Dr. William Dement, an international expert on sleep disorders and director of the Sleep Clinic at Stanford University School of Medicine, explains, "Most physicians dread the arrival of a chronic insomnia patient. If one asks a large group of doctors if any of them enjoy managing chronic insomnia, not a single hand will go up." It is no wonder that the vast majority of cases of insomnia go undiagnosed and untreated!

There is another reason insomniacs can't turn to their doctor for help: medicine has not developed an effective treatment for insomnia. Until recently, the only medical treatments available were sleeping pills such as Halcion, Restoril, Dalmane, Xanax, Ativan, Klonopin, and many others. Sleeping pills, however, are no longer considered a safe or appropriate treatment for chronic insomnia because they can have serious side effects that far outweigh their benefits; are only moderately effective for insomnia and stop working over time; strengthen the belief that the cure for insomnia comes from external factors; and can lead to physical or psychological dependency, which can cause feelings of helplessness, loss of control, and lowered self-esteem.

Most important, *sleeping pills don't cure insomnia, because they don't treat the causes of insomnia.* Consequently, if you rely on sleeping pills, your sleep may improve while you take the pills, but as soon as you stop, your insomnia will return, thereby sustaining the cycle of insomnia and sleeping pills.

Given everything we know about the drawbacks to sleeping pills, why do so many doctors still prescribe them? Partly because when doctors are busy and don't know what to do about insomnia, sleeping pills are a fast and easy solution. Another reason is the pervasive influence of drug companies, which sponsor scientific conferences, advertise in medical journals, send sales personnel to doctors' offices, supply free samples of sleep medications, and fund research studies that pay part of doctors' salaries. Therefore, doctors may be subtly influenced to prescribe the sleeping pills that the drug companies manufacture.

Doctors also prescribe sleeping pills because of the predominant attitude in medicine today that drugs are the best treatment for health problems. This drug-oriented approach, which focuses on treating the body, has worked well for acute and infectious illnesses. However, it has been largely ineffective in the treatment of today's chronic health problems such as stroke, heart disease, arthritis, cancer, insomnia, chronic pain, and mental illness, in which emotional, behavioral, and lifestyle factors play a prominent role.

Psychotherapy and Over-the-Counter Sleep Aids

Not surprisingly, 85 percent of insomniacs never seek medical help. Insomnia has become an epidemic affecting desperate, silent sufferers who, believing that their doctors can't help them or will prescribe habit-forming prescription sleeping pills, have been left to fend for themselves, typically spending years battling the problem futilely and suffering needlessly.

You may be one of the many insomniacs who have turned to expensive, time-consuming psychotherapy in your belief, or perhaps your doctor's, that insomnia is caused by "psychological problems." Not only does this belief induce feelings of helplessness and diminished self-esteem; there also is no scientific proof that psychotherapy is effective for insomnia, in large part because the majority of insomniacs do not have a psychiatric problem such as anxiety or depression. This is why trying to treat insomnia as a problem caused by psychiatric factors is destined to fail and only contributes to the stigma of insomnia being a "psychiatric" problem.

Millions of other insomniacs have turned to a slew of new over-the-counter nighttime sleep aids such as Tylenol PM, Excedrin PM, and Anacin PM, whose manufacturers have capitalized on this epidemic. These products, cloaked in the brand names of trusted medicines, avoid the stigma associated with prescription sleeping pills. Consequently, they are one of the fastest-growing classes of health care products today, with sales soaring to over $100 million in 1992. Yet, in truth, there is no scientific evidence that these medications are any more effective than a sugar pill!

Like prescription sleeping pills, over-the-counter sleeping aids can have unwanted side effects, lose effectiveness over time, and bolster the belief that the cure for insomnia comes from something external, which can foster psychological dependency and feelings of helplessness. Most important, these sleep aids don't cure insomnia because they don't treat the causes. Therefore, if you stop taking over-the-counter sleep aids, your insomnia will return.

Insomniacs have spent an additional $200 million annually on the most recent self-help craze for insomnia: melatonin. Health fads are nothing new, but rarely does one strike with the force of "melatonin madness," which hit its peak in 1995. Advertised at drug stores with signs proclaiming WE HAVE MELATONIN and extolled by the media and national magazines and books as the cure-all for insomnia, melatonin has also been trumpeted as a cure for heart disease, diabetes, depression, and aging. Demand for melatonin was so high that for almost a year vendors had a hard time keeping it in stock.

As we will see, however, the exaggerated claims about melatonin's benefits for insomniacs go far beyond established scientific evidence. It turns out that these claims are based on only a few selected studies, one of which was conducted by a scientist who owns a company that sells melatonin. What insomniacs do not know is that there are just as many studies showing that melatonin has no consistent beneficial effect on insomnia. Consequently, the public has been given an unbalanced picture about the present state of knowledge concerning melatonin, knowledge that is woefully incomplete. Therefore, if you are using melatonin, you are assuming unknown risks.

Why are insomniacs willing to spend money on melatonin and gamble their health on unproven claims about its effects on sleep? Probably because melatonin is available over the counter, is inexpensive, is promoted as "natural" (lead is also natural, yet can be dangerous), and because the lure of a fast and easy panacea for insomnia is irresistible.

Although melatonin may ultimately prove to be effective for some insomniacs, you are risking your health by using it. You are also relying on something external, which only leads to dependency. And because melatonin, like all drugs, does not treat the causes of insomnia, your insomnia will return if you stop taking it.

A Breakthrough in the Treatment of Insomnia

The only true hope for insomnia sufferers is the development of a safe, natural, and effective drug-free treatment that addresses the causes of insomnia. This program has not existed—until now.

Based on ten years of research and clinical practice that I have conducted at Harvard Medical School, the groundbreaking program presented in this book is the *only* drug-free program scientifically proven to conquer insomnia. The results are extraordinary: 100 percent of insomnia patients report improved sleep and 75 percent become normal sleepers as a result of this program; improved sleep is seen to be maintained or even enhanced at long-term follow-up; and insomniacs fall asleep faster using this program than using sleeping pills.

The program is also natural, easy to learn, and practical. It has no side effects, yields results that last, optimizes empowerment and self-control by demonstrating that the cure for insomnia resides within you, enhances mind-body control, and improves health and well-being.

Why This Program Is Different

My insomnia program achieves its remarkable results because it is based on a simple yet powerful concept: *insomnia can only be treated by addressing all the underlying causes.* In most instances, the causes of insomnia are thoughts and behaviors (habits) that are learned and can be unlearned. Some examples include:

- Attitudes and beliefs about sleep
- Negative, stressful thoughts about insomnia
- Feelings of loss of control over sleep
- Inadequate exercise or exposure to sunlight
- Going to bed too early or sleeping too late
- Trying to control sleep rather than letting it occur naturally

- Negative responses to stress
- Lying awake in bed, frustrated and tense

The following story, about one of my patients, illustrates the idea that insomnia is caused by thoughts and behaviors. Does her experience sound familiar?

Carol was a forty-seven-year-old nurse whose insomnia began after the death of a close friend. After experiencing sleeplessness for a few weeks, she started to worry about it, which only made it harder for her to sleep. Carol also began "trying" to fall asleep, which backfired and made her more wide awake, tense, and frustrated.

After a month of sleepless nights, Carol began to expect that she wouldn't sleep, which caused her to fear going to bed. Although Carol had exercised for years, she became so fatigued from insomnia that she stopped exercising. She also began to try to catch up on sleep by spending more time in bed and sleeping late on weekends, all of which seemed to make her sleep worse.

Carol became so desperate that she began drinking a glass of wine or taking a sleeping pill to fall sleep, both of which disturbed the quality of her sleep and made her feel guilty and out of control. Her preoccupation with sleep, coupled with the stress of diminished performance at work, only compounded her insomnia. It wasn't long before Carol began to wonder if something was wrong with her mind and whether she should visit a psychiatrist.

By the time Carol came to see me, she was sleeping less than five hours per night and had been experiencing insomnia for several years. As a result, she always felt exhausted and irritable and was becoming depressed. She perceived her bed as the "enemy" and wondered whether she would ever sleep well again.

Carol then entered my Insomnia Program at Deaconess Hospital. After just a few days in the program, her sleep started to improve. After six weeks, she eliminated sleeping pills, fell asleep easily, and stayed asleep. As a result, she was able to sleep over eight hours per night, awakened refreshed, and "loved her bed again." She also felt more empowered, more confident, and had more control over her mind and body. Even Carol's husband remarked that she was like a new person!

Larry was another patient who came to my program suffering from insomnia. He was a fifty-year-old attorney whose insomnia began during law school. Although Larry could fall asleep easily, he frequently awoke during the night and would lie awake for hours. When Larry came to see me, he had been experiencing insomnia for more than five years and was sleeping about four hours per night, leaving him feeling wiped out, frustrated, and desperate.

After two weeks in my program, Larry slept through the night for the first time in years. By the time he completed the program, he was sleeping nearly seven hours per night and was able to fall asleep again easily if he woke up. Larry was calmer, more energetic, and more productive during the day and also felt more control over his emotions and health.

Carol and Larry achieved their remarkable success by learning a variety of nondrug techniques:

- Viewing insomnia as a learned problem that can be unlearned
- Changing negative, stressful thoughts about sleep
- Managing stress more effectively
- Eliciting the relaxation response, an inborn biological response that allowed them to voluntarily produce the brain-wave patterns that induce sleep
- Using the power and biology of positive beliefs about sleep
- Strengthening the brain's sleep rhythm by reducing excessive time in bed and getting out of bed at the same time every day
- Receiving exposure to bright sunlight and exercising at specific times of the day
- Unlearning the habit of *trying* to sleep

- Using naps to boost mood and performance
- Developing a sense of control over sleep

Carol's and Larry's cases illustrate that insomnia can be conquered only by addressing all the underlying causes, which, in most cases, are thoughts and behaviors. Sleeping pills and psychotherapy don't effectively treat insomnia because they don't treat the thoughts and behaviors that cause insomnia; they reinforce dependency on external solutions, which minimizes self-control and empowerment.

You, too, can improve your sleep and your life the way Carol and Larry did. The rest of this book will show you how.

CHAPTER TWO

Some Basic Facts About Sleep and Insomnia

We spend a notable portion of our lives asleep, yet most of us understand very little about sleep and insomnia. What happens during sleep? What is its purpose? Does sleep change as we age? Are there different kinds of insomnia? And how does insomnia develop?

Unfortunately, our answers to these questions are often based on erroneous information. In this chapter, we will separate fact from fiction by learning some essential facts about sleep and insomnia. Learning about sleep makes it less mysterious, which will give you a feeling of control over insomnia. This knowledge is also a vital prerequisite to understanding and utilizing the drug-free techniques described in the remaining chapters.

Let's begin by investigating what happens during sleep.

The Physiology of Sleep

Five Stages of Sleep

Throughout man's history, sleep was regarded as an inactive state in which our mind and body simply turned off, oblivious to the outer world. In recent decades, with the development of new technology that allows researchers to measure the electrical activity of the brain (called brain wave or EEG recordings), scientists have discovered that sleep is a dynamic state that has an intriguing life of its own.

During a good night's sleep, you close your eyes and first spend a few minutes in a state of relaxed wakefulness that is characterized by drifting thoughts and a brain-wave pattern named alpha. In this state your thoughts gradually wander and your body begins to relax. Next, you drift into Stage 1 sleep, which is a drowsy, relaxed state between waking and sleeping. Here your body becomes still more relaxed: muscle tension lessens, respiration and heart rate slow, body temperature drops, slow, rolling eye movements occur, and a slower brain-wave pattern called theta is generated. You may also experience fragmentary thoughts or a sensation analogous to daydreaming.

When you observe someone "drowsing" during a boring lecture, the person is probably in Stage 1 sleep. However, if awakened from Stage 1, most of us would maintain that we were merely "drifting off" but not actually asleep. Because we are easily awakened from Stage 1, it is not regarded as true sleep.

Following a few minutes in Stage 1, you enter into the first authentic sleep phase, Stage 2. This is deeper than Stage 1, since your body is calmer and you are more detached from the outside world. In this stage, we exhibit brain-wave patterns called sleep spindles and K-complexes, which represent intermittent attempts by the brain to preserve awareness before we "turn off" to our surroundings. Stage 2 is regarded as a light stage of sleep, for we are easily awakened from it.

After about thirty to forty-five minutes in Stage 2, you enter the most profound phases of sleep, Stages 3 and 4. These stages are distinguished by very slow brain-wave patterns named delta and are collectively termed slow-wave sleep, or deep sleep. In these stages, our physiological activity, including respiration, oxygen consumption, heart rate, and blood pressure, realizes its lowest level of the day. It is very difficult to awaken from deep sleep because we are nearly shut off from awareness of the exterior world. Children are particularly unwakeable from deep sleep. If they are awakened from this sleep stage, they will often feel groggy, confused, or disoriented and won't remember it later.

Following about forty-five minutes in deep sleep, we revert to Stage 2 for a few minutes, then enter the visual, emotional world of dream sleep. If awakened during dream sleep, we nearly always describe a dream. Dreams are often detailed, have a continuous quality, and are vivid, bizarre, or sometimes even frightening. Dream sleep is also termed rapid eye movement (REM) sleep, for our eyes move around rapidly while we dream. Although no one knows whether we literally "watch" our dreams, it appears that eye movements do seem to coincide with the actions in our dreams. And contrary to what some people believe, everyone dreams; it's simply that we forget most of them.

The brain and body display significant levels of activity while we dream. For instance, heart rate, blood pressure, and breathing rate escalate and become highly irregular during dreaming; our brain waves also accelerate and blood flow to the brain rises dramatically. In fact, our brain-wave patterns during dream sleep are similar to those that occur when we are awake. For this reason, REM sleep is also called paradoxical sleep.

Another curious finding is that penile erection in males and clitoral engorgement in females also occurs during REM. These changes are probably reflective of the body's general physiological arousal during REM rather than the sexual content of dreams. Penile erection during REM is often used as a test for whether male impotence is physiological or psychological in nature. If erection doesn't occur during REM, the impotence is likely physiological; if it does, psychological factors are more likely to be the problem.

Because REM sleep is such an active period of mental and physiological activity, we are more apt to awaken from this stage and are more likely to feel alert when we do.

Except for small muscle twitches in the face and fingers, we cannot move when we dream because our large body muscles are paralyzed, apparently so that we can't act out our dreams. Thus, REM sleep can be conceived of as an active brain in a paralyzed body.

During a sound night's sleep, we progress from Stage 1 to Stage 4 and then to REM sleep in about ninety minutes. A good sleeper will move through four to six of these ninety-minute sleep cycles during the night, spending about 5 percent of the night in Stage 1, 50 percent in Stage 2, 20 percent in deep sleep, and 25 percent in REM sleep. Whether bedtime is 9:00 P.M., 11:00 P.M., or 1:00 A.M., sleep consistently follows this cyclical pattern.

During the early part of sleep, deep-sleep periods are lengthier, sometimes lasting up to one hour, whereas REM periods last only a few minutes. As the night proceeds, however, deep-sleep periods grow shorter and the duration of REM periods increases so that, by the final sleep cycle, REM periods may persist for an hour. We therefore obtain most of our deep sleep during the first half of the night and the majority of our dream and light sleep in the second half.

Because sleep grows lighter as the night proceeds, awakenings are more prone to occur during the second half of the night. It is also normal to wake up six or more times, particularly when we shift from one sleep stage to another. We normally fall back to sleep within seconds after these awakenings and don't recall them the following morning.

Why Do We Sleep?

We understand a considerable amount about the physiology of sleep. However, the answer to one central question—the precise function of sleep and what it does for our brain and body—remains a puzzle. Even though we spend almost one-third of our lives asleep, there is no one theory about the function of sleep that is accepted by most sleep researchers.

For our distant ancestors, sleep may have served a general survival purpose by forcing them to be inactive at night when their ability to see, find food, and defend themselves against predators was poor. Since our ancestors didn't function well at night, they slept, tucked out of harm's way.

Research on deep sleep suggests that it is a state of profound rest in which the brain and body shut down. Deep sleep also seems to serve a major biological restorative function by renewing our physical energy. Most of the blood in our body is directed to the muscles during deep sleep to help replenish muscular energy. Since most of the blood flow is directed to the muscles during deep sleep, there is little blood flow to the brain, which means that our brain is very inactive. Deep sleep also affords a period of time for our immune system to turn on to combat illnesses. This may explain why we seem to sleep more when we are ill.

Several factors suggest that deep sleep is essential and is the most vital stage. First, deep sleep occurs first during the night and is therefore the stage least likely to be missed. Second, unlike the other stages, we recoup or "make up" virtually all the deep sleep lost as a consequence of sleep deprivation. Third, compared to the other sleep stages, we experience the greatest impairment in our physical functioning (such as aching muscles and stiffness upon awakening) when we forfeit deep sleep.

Stage 2 sleep is probably a less potent form of deep sleep and is also involved with restoring physical energy. However, the brain apparently doesn't regard Stage 2 as important as it does deep sleep, for it does not attempt to recover Stage 2 after sleep loss.

REM sleep is perhaps the most fascinating yet least understood stage. Dreams were viewed by Sigmund Freud as a window to the unconscious and have long been associated with the processing of emotional material. However, contemporary research intimates that a principal function of REM sleep is to permit us to process and save novel information in memory, particularly information learned over the latter portion of each day, and "how to" or procedural memory for activities such as typing, driving, or scuba diving.

One reason newborns occupy much of the day sleeping is that they must spend a substantial amount of time in REM sleep to store all the new information to which they are exposed during the first few months of life. Newborns spend a greater percentage of time in REM sleep compared to adults, and it has been suggested that, in the womb, the fetus may spend all of its time in REM. Because REM is so prominent early in life, some scientists speculate that it plays an important role in the maturation of the brain.

Just as deep sleep seems to be a required stage of sleep, so too does REM sleep. We know this because if we are deprived of REM, we will try to make up for it in the form of REM rebound. Nevertheless, the fact that we make up only about half of the REM sleep that we lose as a consequence of sleep deprivation suggests that it is not as crucial to the brain as deep sleep. And other than causing anxiety, irritability, and difficulty concentrating, there is no proof that REM sleep deprivation causes serious psychological or physical health problems. In fact, as we will explore in chapter 4, deprivation of REM sleep actually improves mood and daytime functioning in some depressed patients.

Now, let's shift to another facet of the physiology of sleep that will be beneficial in understanding and utilizing many of the techniques in this book: the connection between sleep and body temperature.

Body Temperature and Sleep

Though many people think their body temperature remains constant at about 98.6 degrees Fahrenheit, research reveals that it in fact follows a circadian ("about a day") rhythm that varies throughout the day.

Body temperature is lowest in the early morning hours and then commences climbing just before sunrise. It continues to increase until midafternoon and then drops somewhat before rising again and attaining its daily peak around 6:00 P.M. A few hours later, body temperature drops until we fall asleep, then declines more rapidly until it realizes its daily low again at about 4:00 A.M. In a healthy young adult, the variation between the daily minimum and maximum body temperature is about one and a half degrees.

The circadian rhythm of body temperature is closely linked to the variations in our daily levels of activity, alertness, and sleepiness. We are most alert and active when body temperature is highest, which is typically in the late morning and early evening. We grow sleepier and less active as body temperature declines at night, with the strongest desire for sleep occurring at around 3:30 A.M. These daily changes in body temperature and levels of alertness occur regardless of how well we slept the night before, so that, even after sleep loss, we will feel more alert as body temperature rises.

The words *lark* and *owl,* which are sometimes used to characterize persons who attain peaks of alertness and performance at different times of the day, are good examples of the connection between body temperature and alertness. Owls, or night people, function best in the evening because their body temperature peaks later in the day; larks, or morning people, in contrast, are at their optimum earlier in the day because their body temperature rises earlier.

Recent studies have revealed that sleep and body temperature are directly influenced by the daily cycles of sunlight and darkness and their effect on melatonin, a naturally occurring hormone found in the brain. When sunlight enters our eyes, melatonin levels decrease, which signals body temperature to rise. Conversely, when the sun sets, melatonin levels rise, prompting body temperature to decline. Because melatonin production is spurred by darkness, it has been dubbed the vampire hormone. (We'll examine the use of synthetic melatonin as a sleeping pill in chapter 3.)

Two Brain Systems That Govern Sleep

Sleep and wakefulness are also regulated by two systems in the brain: a wakefulness system and a sleep system. For good sleepers, the stronger wakefulness system dominates during the day and keeps us awake for about sixteen hours. After that, the wakefulness system diminishes in strength, and the weaker sleep system becomes dominant and keeps us asleep for about eight hours.

Even while we are deeply asleep, the wakefulness system is operating and evaluating what is occurring around us—the sound of a clock, the temperature of the room, the covers falling off—and can respond to these circumstances. Moreover, this system is more responsive to some things than others, depending upon the significance of what is happening in the immediate environment. Examples include parents who may sleep through a thunderstorm yet wake instantly to the sound of their crying newborn, and people who can awaken within minutes of a certain time without the aid of an alarm clock. We are therefore never altogether oblivious to the outside world, even when deeply asleep.

Some individuals seem to be equipped with a robust sleep system and can sleep "like a log" no matter what happens (much to the frustration of insomniacs!). In contrast, others possess a sleep system that is too weak, or a wakefulness system that is too strong, and thus may be more vulnerable to sleep problems. This is no surprise to parents who have at least two children and have noticed that each has a distinct sleep pattern in terms of how much sleep is required, how easily sleep comes, and how soundly they sleep through the night.

Insomniacs who have been lifelong poor sleepers may have a genetic tendency toward a more temperamental sleep system. However, since learned sleep habits and behaviors play a salient role in perpetuating insomnia, even these people can utilize the techniques in this book to master insomnia.

Sleep Changes As We Age

Our bodies change in many ways as we get older. Sleep is no different. Realizing that changes in sleep are a common part of aging will provide you with a sense of control over sleep and will make it less likely that you will construe these changes as insomnia.

As we age, the amount of sleep we obtain changes. Sleep decreases from about sixteen to eighteen hours a day in newborns to nearly ten hours for ten-year-olds and to approximately eight hours during the teenage years. We sleep about seven hours a night in middle age, and by our seventies sleep time decreases to roughly six and a half hours. However, we compensate by obtaining about an hour of additional sleep in the form of daytime naps.

The most notable age-related change in sleep concerns its quality, which declines in middle age. Specifically, we produce less deep sleep and sleep more lightly (particularly men). We also wake up more frequently and for longer intervals. In fact, by the time we reach our seventies, deep sleep has practically disappeared. As a consequence, we sleep even more lightly and are awakened more easily by internal and external disturbances.

These sleep changes, which are comparable to age-related changes in physical and mental skills, probably reflect natural aging of the brain's sleep system. They are compounded by other stressors frequent among the aged—loneliness, bereavement, concerns about finances, health, or death—and by other medical problems and medications that can interfere with sleep.

Our body-temperature rhythm also changes with age. For instance, the daily variations in body temperature diminish in the elderly (due in part to the fact that they are more likely to cut down on their physical activity and exposure to sunlight), which causes poorer sleep. For reasons not wholly understood, the body temperature of elderly people also starts to rise and fall earlier in the day, resulting in a tendency to fall asleep earlier and wake earlier.

Though these age-related changes in sleep may explain why many older people complain of insomnia, seniors need to understand that insomnia is not an inevitable consequence of aging. Perhaps because changes in sleep are normal, the majority of the elderly seem to adjust favorably to them and don't report insomnia. And for those who do, the behavioral techniques described in this book can be used to surmount the problem.

Now that you have a basic understanding of normal sleep, let's explore and compare some basic facts about insomnia that will also be beneficial in understanding and employing our techniques for overcoming it.

The Various Types of Insomnia

- Suzette turned off the lights at 11:00 P.M. but couldn't fall asleep. For the next few hours, she tossed and turned and finally dozed off around 3:30 A.M. Once asleep, she stayed asleep until her alarm woke her at 7:30 A.M.
- Toby turned off her lights at midnight and, unlike Suzette, fell asleep right away. Nevertheless, Toby woke up after only a few hours and couldn't return to sleep. She tossed and turned for what seemed like hours and finally fell asleep again for a few hours. She woke up at 4:30 A.M. and was unable to get back to sleep.
- Dan has no difficulty falling asleep and does not lie awake during the night. However, his sleep consistently seems unrefreshing, light, and restless, almost as if he

never attains a deep sleep. By morning, Dan feels like he hasn't slept at all.

Suzette, Toby, and Dan personify the three types of insomnia: problems falling asleep, waking up and lying awake during the night or early morning, and poor quality of sleep. Lying awake in bed for an average of half an hour or more before falling asleep is termed sleep-onset insomnia, whereas waking during the night and lying awake for an average of thirty minutes or more is known as sleep-maintenance insomnia.

Studies comprising several thousand insomnia patients have revealed that sleep-onset insomniacs average about an hour and a quarter to fall asleep while sleep-maintenance insomniacs lie awake during the night for a similar amount of time.

You may experience one or a combination of these types of insomnia, or you may discover that your insomnia changes over time from one type to another.

To make a clinical diagnosis of insomnia, it's not merely how long you lie awake or the quantity of sleep that matters; you must also perceive detrimental consequences from disturbed sleep that extend into your day, such as irritability, fatigue, drowsiness, and impaired performance or productivity. Accordingly, if you have trouble falling asleep or staying asleep at night but feel alert and rested during the day, you are *not* an insomniac but a person who just requires less sleep.

How common is insomnia? Probably, it is the most frequent health complaint following pain and headaches. Many studies have established that about one-third of adults experience insomnia. However, a 1995 Harris poll and a 1997 survey by *Consumer Reports* found that the percentage of adults complaining of sleep difficulties has increased to one-half. Studies also indicate that about half of the adults who report insomnia endure it on a regular, chronic basis. Consequently, you can take some solace in knowing that, if you are lying awake at night, millions of other adults are too.

Insomnia affects people from all walks of life, but it is more frequent among women and the elderly. We have already examined several reasons the elderly are more prone to insomnia, but why women? We do not know for certain, but it may be that women are simply more likely or willing to acknowledge that they experience insomnia. It is also conceivable that, for middle-aged women, the psychological and hormonal changes associated with menopause may precipitate insomnia.

The Physiology of Insomnia

Numerous studies employing brain-wave recordings have corroborated that the sleep of insomniacs differs from normal sleepers in a number of ways: insomniacs require longer to fall asleep, sleep more lightly, wake up more frequently and for longer periods during the night, and sleep fewer hours. We have also discovered some significant information about the physiology of insomnia that may explain why insomniacs sleep poorly. For instance, insomniacs have greater physical tension during the night compared to good sleepers as indicated by faster heart rate and more muscle tension.

In my research, I established that insomniacs have faster brain-wave patterns in bed than good sleepers, which is consonant with heightened mental activity. Subsequent chapters will examine how this program slows brain waves and curbs this mental activity, thereby improving sleep.

The most recent investigations on the physiology of insomnia pertain to disruptions in the circadian rhythm of body temperature. Several studies have determined that insomniacs display smaller increases and decreases in their daily body-temperature rhythm relative to good sleepers. This "flattening" of the body-temperature rhythm may be due to the fact that many insomniacs reduce their physical activity because they feel fatigued. This pattern reinforces a cycle of fatigue, diminished physical activity, and increased insomnia.

Other studies have also revealed that the body temperature of sleep-onset insomniacs starts to drop about three hours later at night than normal sleepers, making it more difficult to fall asleep. Additional studies have shown that the body temperature of sleep-maintenance insomniacs doesn't drop as much during the night as normal sleepers, which makes it difficult to sleep deeply. In subsequent chapters, you will learn a number of techniques that improve sleep by normalizing these disruptions in the body-temperature rhythm.

Collectively, the research on the physiology of insomnia suggests that insomniacs have improperly balanced sleep and wakefulness systems: the former is too weak, the latter too strong, and sleep is too easily disturbed. Another way to think about this is that, on some nights, your sleep system is just not ready for sleep. Thus, you are more likely to lie awake. And what happens when you lie awake? You think, which further stimulates your wakefulness system. Therefore, the "racing mind" that you may experience is sometimes the *result* of lying awake, not the cause; and blaming insomnia on being unable to "turn off my mind," which is routine among insomniacs and which escalates feelings of loss of control, is not always accurate.

An important concept to which we will return repeatedly is that the techniques in this program function by teaching you to enhance your sleep system and set the stage for sleep to occur. Consequently, your sleep system will be less temperamental and you will sleep more effortlessly. You will also realize that you can attain greater control over your body and your sleep than you ever imagined.

How Chronic Insomnia Evolves

Occasional bouts of insomnia are normal and inevitable reactions to significant life events such as losses like death or divorce; family or work-related stressors; health problems, hospitalizations, or recovery from surgery; and relationship changes. Insomnia is such a customary reaction to these stressful life events (only 5 percent of adults report that they have never experienced insomnia) that some sleep experts surmise insomnia may serve an adaptive purpose in that it compels us to spend extra time thinking about and coping with these stressors.

Fortunately, this type of insomnia, called short-term insomnia, typically persists for only a few days or weeks, and once the precipitating stressor fades or we have adjusted to it, life and sleep revert to normal.

For some individuals, however, insomnia takes on a life of its own and persists long after the initial precipitating event has been resolved. This type of insomnia, which endures for a month or longer, is termed chronic. It may affect you a few nights a week or almost nightly. Also, chronic insomnia can occur every week or in a cyclical fashion, being worse in some weeks than others. It frequently lasts for years, as illustrated by the finding that my patients have experienced insomnia for an average of ten years by the time they come to me.

Why does short-term insomnia develop into chronic insomnia for some people but not others? Because some individuals react to short-term insomnia by worrying about sleep loss. After a few weeks of lying awake at night, frustrated and anxious about insomnia, they start to anticipate not sleeping and become apprehensive about going to bed. They soon learn to associate the bed with sleeplessness and frustration; consequently, the bed quickly becomes a learned cue for wakefulness and insomnia.

In an attempt to cope with insomnia, most insomniacs begin to engage in an assortment of behaviors, or habits, that may seem to help in the short run but actually sustain insomnia. Here are some examples that will undoubtedly sound familiar:

- Going to bed earlier, sleeping later (especially on weekends), and spending more time in bed in an effort to "catch up" on sleep
- Trying to control or "force" sleep in the belief that "If I try just a little harder, sleep is bound to come"
- Attempting to relax in bed by reading or watching television
- Taking naps
- Using alcohol to promote sleep or caffeine to combat the daytime fatigue produced by insomnia
- Reducing physical activity and exercise because of the fatigue caused by insomnia

Daily stress also exacerbates poor sleep, particularly on very stressful days or during stressful periods of time, and impairs the ability to cope with insomnia. You will learn more about how to improve sleep by managing stress in part III.

Now you should understand how the combination of worry about sleep, maladaptive sleep habits, and daytime stress can transform a brief period of insomnia into a case of learned chronic insomnia that has a life of its own. When I explain this model of chronic insomnia to my patients, their usual response is, "That sounds exactly like me!"

An important aspect of this model is that, although a number of factors may initially cause insomnia, treatment of chronic insomnia must focus not on the precipitating factors but on changing the thoughts and behaviors that play the main role in perpetuating insomnia. Since these thoughts and behaviors are learned, they can also be "unlearned," using the techniques I will describe.

In subsequent chapters you will perform your own assessment of the thoughts and behaviors that disturb your sleep, and you will learn more about how these thoughts and behaviors produce chronic insomnia. Most important, you will learn a variety of drug-free techniques designed to effectively change the thoughts and behaviors that are disrupting your sleep.

Do medical problems cause chronic insomnia? Yes, they can cause short-term insomnia and can contribute to disturbed sleep in chronic insomniacs; however, thoughts and behaviors, not medical problems, play the primary role in most cases of chronic insomnia.

What about depression, anxiety, and other mental health problems in chronic insomnia? It is true that insomnia is a frequent symptom of many psychiatric disorders such as depression and anxiety. It is also true that insomniacs tend to exhibit higher levels of depression and anxiety compared to normal sleepers. Research I have conducted, however, suggests that insomnia patients do not have greater levels of anxiety or depression than patients with other chronic health complaints such as headaches, pain, gastrointestinal problems, infertility, and hypertension or heart disease. Studies also document that the majority of patients who visit their doctor with a main complaint of chronic insomnia do not have a diagnosable psychiatric disorder such as depression or anxiety. For those insomnia patients who do, research has shown that, for some of these individuals, depression can be the consequence of insomnia, not the cause. Additionally, because thoughts and behaviors almost always cause chronic insomnia, the techniques I offer are appropriate as an adjunctive treatment to drug therapy or psychotherapy for insomnia patients with depression or anxiety.

I have a major, primary concern about insomnia—the tendency for both insomniacs and health professionals to conceptualize insomnia as a psychiatric problem. In truth, this is erroneous, as exemplified by the fact that there is not one scientific study demonstrating that psychotherapy is effective in treating chronic insomnia. Regarding insomnia as a psychiatric problem just reinforces the stigma associated with insomnia and diminishes self-esteem and confidence.

To return to my central theme: insomnia can be overcome only by addressing its underlying causes, which, in most cases, are thoughts and behaviors. This program has achieved its extraordinary results because it effectively changes these habits. At the same time, it optimizes empowerment and self-control by demonstrating that the key to conquering insomnia resides within *you*.

CHAPTER THREE

Putting Sleeping Pills to Rest

Just a few years ago, doctors dispensed sleeping pills as if they were candy. Today, sleeping pills are increasingly recognized as only a short-term solution that can evolve into a long-term problem. Why? Because, as we will explore in this chapter, regular use of sleeping pills is no longer considered safe or appropriate due to their undesirable and potentially dangerous side effects. Furthermore, sleeping pills are only moderately effective for insomnia and don't help insomniacs become normal sleepers.

Sleeping pills also fail to treat the causes of insomnia. Because they treat only insomnia's symptoms, any improvement in sleep can only be temporary, thereby perpetuating the cycle of insomnia and sleeping pills. Ironically, many people initially turn to sleeping pills because insomnia has left them feeling helpless and out of control. However, sleeping pills can become a trap that escalates feelings of dependency, lowered self-esteem, and guilt. You end up having to cope with two stressful problems: insomnia *and* dependency on sleeping pills.

Recently, increased awareness of the many drawbacks associated with sleeping pills has led to a significant decline in their use. The number of sleeping-pill prescriptions has dropped over the past twenty years by about two-thirds, from 60 million in 1970 to about 20 million in 1990.

Yet despite the fact that the nondrug techniques described in this program have been scientifically proven to be effective in treating insomnia, recent studies indicate that physicians still consider sleeping pills to be the most effective treatment and continue to overprescribe them. And while use of prescription sleeping pills has declined, use of over-the-counter preparations such as Tylenol PM, Excedrin PM, and melatonin has risen dramatically in the 1990s.

As a result, many insomniacs have become trapped in the cycle of insomnia and dependency on sleeping pills. In fact, over two-thirds of the insomnia patients who come to me are taking sleeping pills at least a few nights a week. Most of these patients are aware of the drawbacks of pills and prefer nondrug approaches to managing insomnia, but they don't know how to escape the sleeping-pill trap.

Sarah was an insomniac enmeshed in the sleeping-pill trap. Her story, unfortunately, is all too common.

Sarah never experienced sleep problems until she underwent surgery for breast cancer. The stress of her surgery, combined with her postoperative pain, caused significant sleep problems during her hospital stay. Therefore, Sarah's doctor prescribed Xanax for her on a nightly basis, which worked nicely in helping her to sleep and to feel less anxious during the day.

After Sarah was discharged from the hospital, her pain subsided but the stress of the surgery continued to disturb her sleep. Sarah's doctor continued to prescribe Xanax, telling her that it was "safe," so Sarah continued taking it every night. About one month later, she noticed that Xanax wasn't working as well; she was having more difficulty falling asleep and continued to wake during the night. When Sarah told her doctor, he advised her to increase her use of Xanax to two tablets per night. It wasn't long before two tablets weren't working and Sarah had to increase the dose to three tablets a night.

At this point, Sarah knew she was becoming addicted to Xanax, so she tried to go without it for a few days. Unfortunately, this exacerbated her insomnia and she felt she had no choice but to resume the medication. Eventually, she reached the point at which, if she didn't take four Xanax tablets at bedtime, she could not sleep at all. Sarah also noticed a hangover effect from the medication that was impairing her thinking and coordination in the morning.

By the time Sarah came to see me, she had been taking four Xanax tablets every night for four years! Her memory was becoming poorer and she viewed herself as an addict. Sarah was also experiencing significant guilt and lowered self-esteem about her sleeping-pill dependency; she felt hopeless, out of control. Even her doctor was desperate and didn't know what to do for her.

As Sarah's story illustrates, you can't buy sleep or solve chronic insomnia with a sleeping pill. Although sleeping pills can be effective for the management of short-term insomnia, they are only moderately effective in helping insomniacs fall asleep. Sleeping pills also become increasingly ineffective with regular use and can cause many side effects, such as dependency, that far outweigh their moderate benefits. From an economic perspective, regular use of sleeping pills can also get expensive; the pills and the visits to the prescribing doctor can end up costing thousands of dollars.

Even if the ideal sleeping pill were developed—one that had no side effects and that produced natural sleep—it would still reinforce the belief that the cure for insomnia comes from something external, and it wouldn't treat the causes of insomnia, which are thoughts and behaviors. So if you rely on a sleeping pill, your sleep may improve while you take it, but insomnia will return as soon as you stop.

In this chapter, we'll take a close look at the three types of sleeping pills—benzodiazepines, antidepressants, and over-the-counter products—and their effectiveness, side effects, differences, and other issues associated with their use. We will also look at situations when sleeping pills may be appropriate and will explore clinically proven techniques for putting sleeping pills to rest for good.

Benzodiazepines

In the 1970s, sleeping pills were the most widely prescribed medications in the world. They still represent big business for pharmaceutical companies, accounting for a whopping $400 million in annual sales. The most frequently prescribed sleeping pills, called benzodiazepines (BZs), are much safer than the older sleeping pills, called barbiturates, which had a much greater potential for addiction and overdose. (Marilyn Monroe died from an overdose of barbiturates.)

Although some BZs are marketed as sleeping pills, most are actually sold as antianxiety drugs. Although this may seem odd, it is done for economic reasons: the companies that manufacture antianxiety drugs do not want to spend the additional millions of dollars necessary to test and market them as sleeping pills. In fact, physicians routinely prescribe antianxiety drugs as sleeping pills.

BZs promote sleep by depressing the activity of the brain and slowing brain waves. They reduce the time required to fall asleep, decreasing the number and duration of nighttime awakenings and increasing total sleep time. However, their effectiveness is only moderate. After reviewing nine studies that used sleeping pills to treat insomnia, researchers found that insomniacs still took forty-six minutes to fall asleep after treatment with sleeping pills. So the belief that sleeping pills help insomniacs to fall asleep quickly and cure insomnia is a myth.

BZs also work by clouding our thinking and memory after we take them, which causes us to forget that we are awake during the night. This alteration in the perception of whether or not we are awake explains why insomniacs who take sleeping pills overestimate how long they have slept compared to actual brain-wave recordings. This altered sleep perception also reinforces the belief that sleeping pills are effective, which encourages continued use.

All BZs are about equally effective in inducing sleep. However, they differ in terms of their half-life (the time it takes for the body to break down and eliminate half of the drug taken). Some BZs have a short half-life, meaning that the body gets rid of them quickly, while others stay in the body much longer. In general, BZs with a short half-life are a better choice as sleeping pills since, as we will explore, BZs with a longer half-life can cause next-day drowsiness and adversely affect daytime performance.

Below are many of the commonly prescribed BZs, listed by the brand name, generic name, recommended dosage, and half-life:

BRAND NAME	GENERIC NAME	DOSE (MG/DAY)	HALF-LIFE
Valium	diazepam	5–10	2–5 days
Klonopin	clonazepam	0.5–2	2–3 days
Tranxene	clorazepate	3.75–15	2–4 days
Prosom	estazolam	1–2	8–24 hours
Ativan	lorazepam	1–4	10–20 hours
Xanax	alprazolam	0.5	7–27 hours
Serax	oxazepam	15–30	8–12 hours
Doral	quazepam	7.5–15	2–5 days
Restoril	temazepam	15–30	10–20 hours
Halcion	triazolam	0.125–0.25	2–5 hours
Ambien	zolpidem	5–10	1.5–4.5 hours
Dalmane	flurazepam	15–30	1–5 days

Although BZs may be moderately effective in the short term, sooner or later all lose their effectiveness entirely. This is because, with their continued use, the brain becomes accustomed, or "habituated," to their effects. Indeed, there is no scientific evidence that BZs work for more than four to six weeks of nightly use, hence the reason the National Institutes of Health advise that BZs should not be prescribed for more than two to three weeks at a time. Yet, surprisingly, BZs are routinely prescribed by physicians for months or even years! To make matters worse, several studies have documented that BZ prescriptions are renewed too easily, are not monitored appropriately, and are often written for six-month periods without any follow-up; and patients often exceed the recommended dose.

Regular use of BZs can also result in these other problems, some of them potentially serious:

1. BZs lessen your deep sleep and REM sleep and increase your Stage 2 sleep; consequently, you may fall asleep faster and stay asleep more easily during the night but your sleep will be lighter and of poorer quality.

2. BZs can produce a hangover effect the following day. Although you may not be aware of this effect, it can impair coordination (including the ability to drive a car), alertness, memory, and thinking. The potential for this effect is greater for the elderly, whose bodies do not get rid of medications as quickly, and with medications that have longer half-lives, such as Dalmane. (In fact, if you take Dalmane every night, you may experience a daily hangover effect because you never entirely eliminate it from your body.)

Although people take a sleeping pill to ensure that they will function adequately the next day, there is no evidence to support this assumption. In fact, the daytime hangover effect from a BZ is often worse than the impairment caused by insomnia. Numerous studies have demonstrated that performance of tasks such as driving, adding numbers, playing video games, copying drawings, making decisions, and remembering words is never better after nights when sleeping pills were taken than after nights of poor sleep. So it's a myth that taking a sleeping pill will help you to function better the next day.

Keep in mind that the later you take a BZ (e.g., 3:30 A.M. rather than 11:00 P.M.), the longer these hangover effects will extend into your day. Therefore, if you can't sleep and feel that you must take a sleeping pill in the middle of the night, make sure it's one with a short half-life.

3. If you take a BZ often enough, in large enough doses, and for a long enough time, you can become physically dependent upon it and may experience withdrawal symptoms such as nervousness, headaches, or even seizures if you attempt to stop taking the medication, especially if you stop abruptly. Therefore, BZ dosage should always be reduced gradually.

4. Even though most insomniacs who use BZs never really become physically dependent on the medication, many habitual users become psychologically dependent on the pills. In other words, these individuals believe they cannot fall asleep without a sleeping pill, which causes increased anxiety and insomnia if they attempt to stop taking the medication.

5. With regular use of a BZ, you may develop tolerance to it. Therefore, you will need larger doses for the drug to work, which can result in a never-ending pattern of tolerance, escalating dosage, and greater potential for other side effects.

6. Once your brain has learned to rely on a BZ, you may experience "rebound insomnia" if you attempt to stop the medication. This temporary insomnia (lasting seven to ten days), which can be worse than the insomnia that originally led you to take the sleeping pill, can cause severe anxiety. This anxiety is extremely powerful in strengthening the belief that you cannot sleep without a pill and increases the likelihood that you will resume using the pill and eventually become drug-dependent.

All of these BZ side effects are more likely the larger the dose and more frequently taken, and if you use a BZ for more than a few weeks. Studies on Ambien, a relatively new sleep medication that is similar to but not actually a BZ, indicate that Ambien is less likely than BZs to disturb deep sleep and REM sleep or to produce withdrawal effects or rebound insomnia; it may therefore be a better choice as a sleeping pill. However, Ambien can also lead to physical or psychological dependency.

As if these potential side effects are not enough, there are others: some people experience dizziness, nausea, blurred vision, restlessness, digestive upset, high blood pressure, anxiety, weakness, loss of appetite, and frequent urination after taking a BZ. BZs can also slow down your breathing and exacerbate snoring. Therefore, you should not take these pills if you snore or have sleep apnea (a disorder that we will explore in the next chapter). Although the risk of death from overdose of a BZ is quite small, it increases dramatically when you combine BZs with alcohol. *Never mix alcohol and sleeping pills—if you do, you are risking your life.*

BZs can also have undesirable interactions with other types of medications, so be certain your physician knows about all the medications you are taking. Just as many drugs can endanger a fetus and cause birth defects, so too can BZs. If a pregnant mother is addicted to sleeping pills, her baby can be born addicted and can undergo withdrawal symptoms. Therefore, pregnant or breast-feeding women or those of child-bearing age who are not using birth control methods should *never* use sleeping pills. One final word of caution: if you have a history of addiction to alcohol, nicotine, or caffeine, stay away from sleeping pills, for you are more prone to becoming addicted to them.

The use of BZs by the elderly can be a real problem. As we explored in the previous chapter, older people are more prone to sleep difficulties. Consequently, they are more likely to use sleeping pills than any other age group. However, the elderly are less able to metabolize sleep medications and therefore are more sensitive to the effects and side effects of these drugs, including impaired coordination and driving, a greater risk of falls and fractures, and a greater likelihood of becoming dependent on sleeping pills. Furthermore, older people often take medications for other health problems that can heighten the effects of sleeping pills, so they need to be particularly cautious about combining sleeping pills with other types of medication.

Sleeping pills are overused and abused by many of the elderly. A report from the Pennsylvania Department of Aging, for example, revealed that 85 percent of old people taking sleeping pills were taking too high a dose and 70 percent were taking them for more than the recommended duration. Other studies have uncovered an even more alarming danger of sleeping-pill use by the elderly: it is one of the strongest predictors of nursing home placement because it can lead to a syndrome of daytime drowsiness, amnesia, apathy, and confusion that can mimic dementia or Alzheimer's disease.

Prescribing practices for sleeping pills in nursing homes are also alarming. Several studies have documented that sleeping pills are overly and improperly prescribed in nursing homes and are often given on a routine basis or as a chemical restraint to sedate patients because of staff shortages. (In one study, 95 percent of nursing home residents were prescribed sleeping pills!) Consequently, many nursing home patients muddle through the day, lethargic and tired or even in a drugged daze.

For these reasons, it is essential that older people be extremely cautious about using sleeping pills. Current guidelines suggest that the elderly should take half the usual adult dose of a sleeping pill and never for more than a few weeks. The elderly also need to understand that sleeping pills do not reverse age-related changes in sleep and that the best strategy to deal with these changes is to learn and practice the nondrug techniques described in this book.

Antidepressants

As the name implies, antidepressant medications were developed to treat depression. Some antidepressants such as Prozac (which is presently being taken by millions of Americans) have an energizing effect and can cause insomnia. Therefore, if you are taking Prozac, ask your physician about whether it may be exacerbating your insomnia.

Interestingly, other antidepressants taken in very small doses, such as Elavil, Sinequan, and Desyrel, produce sedation and drowsiness as a side effect. For this reason, physicians are increasingly prescribing small doses of these sedating antidepressants as a sleeping pill for nondepressed individuals who suffer from insomnia.

Like BZs, sedating antidepressants help insomniacs to fall asleep faster, stay asleep, and sleep for longer periods of time. However, even low doses of these medications can cause daytime hangover and lead to psychological dependency. Some people seem to develop tolerance to their effects. They can also cause side effects such as dry mouth, constipation, blurred vision, and urinary problems. And, like BZs, antidepressants can harm a fetus and adversely interact with other medications; *they should never be combined with alcohol.*

Compared to BZs, low-doze sedating antidepressants offer two major advantages: they do not disrupt deep sleep and they do not produce physical dependence or rebound insomnia. For these reasons, many physicians are now choosing to prescribe these medications for insomnia instead of BZs. If you are taking BZs, ask your doctor whether a low-dose sedating antidepressant might be a better sleeping medication for you.

Over-the-Counter Products

The active ingredient in over-the-counter sleep aids (OTCs) is the same antihistamine found in cold and allergy medications such as Benadryl. Because antihistamines produce drowsiness as a side effect, they are also marketed as sleep-promoting agents. This marketing strategy certainly works, for insomniacs spend over $100 million annually on OTCs.

Until recently, the only available OTCs were medications such as Sominex, Unisom, Sleep-Eze, and Nytol. However, since the early 1990s, most of the companies that market analgesics have also sold nighttime sleep aids such as Tylenol PM, Bufferin Nitetime, Anacin PM, and Excedrin PM. Although these products are nothing more than an analgesic combined with an antihistamine, they have resulted in record sales of OTCs, in large part because they avoid the stigma of sleeping pills.

Despite all the advertising claims made for OTCs, there is virtually no scientific evidence that they are more effective than a sugar pill. They may cause drowsiness, but they are not very effective at putting insomniacs to sleep. Indeed, they have the opposite effect of increasing anxiety in some people. The many side effects include daytime sedation, disturbance of REM sleep, tolerance, and psychological dependence.

Synthetic Melatonin

As noted in the previous chapter, melatonin is a naturally occurring brain hormone that plays a role in sleep. Synthetic melatonin has recently been marketed and publicized as a "natural" sleeping pill. However, because melatonin is sold as a "health supplement," it is not regulated by the Food and Drug Administration and there is no assurance of its purity.

Despite all the media hype about melatonin, there has been very little sound scientific research done on this product. Some research indicates that it may be useful for jet lag and perhaps as a sleep aid for elderly insomniacs who produce low levels of natural melatonin. However, there is little if any scientific evidence to support the claim that melatonin is effective for insomnia in young and middle-age adults.

Although several studies found that melatonin was effective for promoting sleep, the studies used normal sleepers, not insomniacs. In the few studies that utilized insomniacs, the results have been inconsistent. Several studies found that melatonin did not significantly improve total sleep time or reduce the time it took to fall asleep. And, in a 1997 survey by *Consumer Reports*, half of the insomniacs who tried melatonin said that it was not helpful.

After reviewing the existing research on the use of melatonin as a sleeping pill, a 1996 National Institutes of Health melatonin workshop urged skepticism. The scientists who participated in this workshop found that many of the studies on melatonin had been poorly conducted, and other scientists were concerned about melatonin's side effects. It may constrict blood vessels and therefore should not be used by those with heart problems. In high doses, melatonin also inhibits fertility and should therefore not be used by women who are trying to conceive. (In fact, melatonin is being tested widely in the Netherlands as a contraceptive; ironically, sleepiness is not a commonly reported side effect, which casts further doubt on its use as a sleeping pill.)

We also know nothing about melatonin's long-term effects on the reproductive and immune systems. Several internationally respected sleep experts have summarized the research on the use of melatonin as a sleeping pill by concluding that it has little value in the treatment of insomnia.

When Sleeping Pills May Be Appropriate

Like most medicines, sleeping pills can be of value if they are used judiciously. Occasional use of a sleeping pill for a few nights or even a few weeks may be appropriate if sleep is temporarily disturbed by jet lag or a stressful event such as the death of a loved one, separation, divorce, or a medical problem. In these circumstances, sleeping pills may help prevent short-term insomnia from evolving into chronic insomnia.

Some sleep experts also believe that keeping a *small* supply of sleeping pills in the medicine cabinet can be helpful for some insomniacs because the knowledge that a sleeping pill is available provides a sense of security and minimizes the fear of insomnia. Other experts maintain that short-term use of sleeping pills may also be appropriate to break the cycle of anxiety and disturbed sleep in severe, chronic insomnia.

No matter what the circumstances, however, you should always attempt to change the thoughts and behaviors that are causing insomnia before you resort to a pill, for if you take sleeping pills you may not have the self-control to use them occasionally and therefore risk becoming dependent upon them. This is the reason many sleep experts recommend against ever using sleeping pills and why the National Institutes of Health state that the treatment of insomnia should always start with behavioral techniques.

If you cannot sleep and choose to take a sleeping pill, you will minimize the likelihood of side effects and dependence if you follow these guidelines:

- Use the nondrug techniques described in this book in conjunction with sleeping pills so that you can taper off their use more quickly
- Use the smallest possible dose of a sleeping pill and do not use it for more than two or three weeks
- Use sleeping pills intermittently, only after two consecutive bad nights of sleep, and never on consecutive nights; this will ensure that you do not use sleep medication more than twice a week
- Never escalate the dose or take a dose higher than your physician has prescribed, and always try to use sleep medications with a short half-life

You Can Put Sleeping Pills to Rest—Permanently

Now you understand the major problems with sleeping pills: people begin by taking them only a few nights a week but often end up taking them much more frequently. Additionally, tolerance often develops to the effects of sleeping pills, and attempts to stop taking them can result in increased anxiety, rebound insomnia, and resumption of use. Ultimately, this trap results in chronic sleeping-pill use that persists for years and causes psychological dependency and feelings of loss of control.

Fortunately, if you are taking sleeping pills, you can learn to escape the sleeping-pill trap. As part of my insomnia program, I have developed and tested techniques that are specifically designed to help you reduce and eliminate sleeping-pill use. In fact, 90 percent of my patients who were taking sleeping pills when they began the program used thee techniques to reduce or eliminate sleeping pills by the end of the program. Indeed, many of my patients have used these techniques to conquer sleeping pills in only a few weeks!

There are two important elements underlying the success of these medication-reduction techniques. First, they are self-paced, so that you can reduce sleeping-pill use at a rate with which you are comfortable. Second, these techniques allow you to decrease your medication gradually rather than abruptly, which can backfire and cause increased anxiety and insomnia. Since regular users of sleeping pills can experience withdrawal symptoms or rebound insomnia if they terminate sleeping-pill use abruptly, gradually tapering off also minimizes the likelihood of these problems. It is also a good idea to discuss these tapering guidelines with your doctor.

Here are the techniques that will enable you escape the sleeping pill trap:

1. Start the medication-reduction techniques when you begin the six-week program described in chapters 5 through 10. As you successfully implement this program, your sleep will improve and you will find that you simply won't need to take a sleeping pill as often. Do not start medication reduction when your life is exceptionally hectic or stressful, and tell someone close to you that you are implementing these techniques; the social support will make it easier.

2. Begin by cutting your dose in half on one of the nights that you take medication. Choose an easy night (such as a weekend night) when there is little pressure and few work obligations the following day and therefore less apprehension about daytime functioning.

3. Once you are sleeping reasonably well on this reduced-dosage night (this may happen right away or may take a few weeks), you will feel more confident about reducing sleep medication and should therefore cut your dose in half on two of the nights that you take medication. Once again, pick an "easy" night and space the reduction nights apart so that, if you do not sleep as well on these nights, you won't experience disturbed sleep two nights in a row.

4. Continue in this fashion until you have cut the dose in half on all the nights that you take sleep medication (obviously you will eventually have to cut the dose in half on consecutive nights, but by then your confidence about reducing the medication will be greatly enhanced). Avoid at all costs going back to the original dose.

5. After you have cut your dose in half on all the nights you take medication, eliminate the remaining half-dose in the same gradual fashion: on one night a week, then two nights, and so on until you are completely medication free. If you are taking multiple medications, use these techniques to get off one first, then work on reducing the second medication.

6. Keep in mind that people who have used sleeping pills in large doses or for long periods of time, or those who are using multiple sleep medications, will naturally require more time to successfully implement these medication-reduction techniques. If you cannot successfully do so yourself, it may be necessary to enlist the assistance of a behavioral psychologist or a sleep disorders center.

7. To reinforce your progress, you will keep a record of your progress in the daily 60-Second Sleep Diary that you will begin in the next chapter and on the Weekly Progress Summary that you will begin in chapter 5.

8. Finally, research on phobias and panic attacks demonstrates that the only way to overcome anxiety-producing situations is to face these situations head-on rather than avoiding them. So the longer you avoid reducing your sleep medication, the more anxious you will be about it.

If you follow these medication-reduction guidelines, you can overcome your dependency on sleeping pills as many of my patients have. Sondra did; here is her story.

Sondra had been a poor sleeper her entire life. Her mother recalled that, even as a baby, Sondra could not fall asleep on her own. By the time Sondra was an adult, she had developed regular, chronic insomnia, typically lying awake for hours during the night.

After the birth of Sondra's first son and his frequent awakenings during the night, Sondra's insomnia became worse. Months later, when her son was finally sleeping through the night, Sondra still found herself waking repeatedly and lying awake for hours.

Sondra and her husband had just started their own business and Sondra felt that her disturbed sleep was seriously impairing her job performance. So she asked her doctor for some sleeping pills. When she assured her doctor that she would take them only once in a while, when she really needed them, he agreed and prescribed Ativan.

Initially, Sondra used Ativan only once a week. However, when she found that it helped her sleep seven hours a night, Sondra took Ativan more frequently. Within six months, she was using it five nights per week. Sondra did not like some of Ativan's side effects, such as morning grogginess, moodiness, and headaches, but she now believed that sleeping pills were the only way for her to get a good night's sleep.

As is often the case, Sondra eventually developed tolerance to Ativan: some nights it would help her sleep six hours, but on other nights she slept only three. Because Sondra feared that her insomnia would get worse if she stopped Ativan, she continued its use.

After five years of using Ativan five nights a week, Sondra finally realized she had to stop using sleeping pills and decided to see me. Why? Sondra and her husband wanted to attempt a second pregnancy and she knew that using sleeping pills during pregnancy could endanger the fetus.

When Sondra began my insomnia program, she practiced the guidelines for reducing sleeping pills. During the first week of the program, she cut her Ativan dose in half. During the second week, she took Ativan on only three nights. By the fourth week of the program, medication was used on only two nights, and by the fifth week, she had achieved seven straight days without a sleeping pill—the first time in over five years!

One week later, Sondra quit using sleeping pills entirely and, to her surprise, was getting the best sleep in years. Within a month, she was sleeping eight hours a night and was confident and relaxed about her sleep. She was amazed at her ability to stop using sleep medication so easily, felt more energetic and productive at work, and looked at herself with a heightened sense of self-esteem. And the biggest benefit of all: Sondra and her husband successfully conceived their second child, who was born only one year after Sondra finished my program.

You, too, can use these techniques to conquer sleeping pills and escape the sleeping-pill trap. You will also accomplish something more fundamental and powerful: you will prove to yourself that you have the power to change your thoughts and behaviors. This power will enhance your self-esteem and you will view yourself in a new way. You will also empower yourself with the knowledge that you can achieve greater control of your body and your health.

In short, conquering sleeping pills can be a catalyst for gaining command of your life.

CHAPTER FOUR

Conducting Your Own Insomnia Self-Assessment

In this chapter, you will cultivate your sense of control over sleep by conducting your own insomnia self-assessment. This assessment, which is the same one I conduct with my patients, is invaluable in learning to conquer insomnia, for it will assist you in evaluating your present sleep pattern, identifying your particular thoughts and behaviors that are causing insomnia, and determining if medical or mental health problems may be contributing to your insomnia.

By conducting your own insomnia self-assessment, you will increase your awareness and understanding of the thoughts and behaviors causing your insomnia. This will help you cultivate a greater sense of control over your sleep. You will feel more relaxed and empowered and will sleep better as a result. Then, in the chapters that follow, we will investigate how these thoughts and behaviors cause insomnia and examine step-by-step techniques for changing these habits.

Determining Your Baseline Sleep Pattern

The first step in conducting your insomnia self-assessment is to accurately establish your current sleep pattern, or what is called your *baseline* sleep pattern.

First, you will need to complete the sleep diary on the following page for seven consecutive mornings. I call this the 60-Second Sleep Diary because it will require only about one minute of your time to fill out each morning when you get out of bed. Take a few moments to review the 60-Second Sleep Diary; it is the same diary used by my patients. (You will need to make seven copies of the diary.)

Most of the items on the 60-Second Sleep Diary are very straightforward. However, three require some additional explanation that will make it easier for you to complete the diary each morning.

1. If you fill out the diary on Monday morning, write "Sunday" in the space marked "night"; if you fill it out on Friday morning, write Thursday in the space marked "night," and so on.
2. Question 7: record the number of hours you allotted for sleep by determining the number of hours elapsed between the time you turned the lights off to go to sleep (question 1) and the time you got out of bed (question 5). For example, if you turned the lights off at 11:00 P.M. and got out of bed at 7:00 A.M., you allotted eights hours for sleep.
3. Question 9: record the dose and the number of prescription or over-the-counter sleeping pills that you took before going to sleep or during the night.

Keep in mind that the 60-Second Sleep Diary is *not* meant to promote clock-watching. If you are overly concerned about how long it took you to fall asleep or how long you were awake during the

60-SECOND SLEEP DIARY

Night ________________ Date ________________

1. Last night, what time did you get into bed? ________________
   Turn the lights off? ________________
2. About how long did it take you to fall asleep? ________________
   ____
3. About how many times did you awaken during the night? ______
   ____
4. For each awakening, about how long were you awake? ________
   1st ________________ 2nd ________________
   3rd ________________ 4th ________________
5. What time was your final wake-up this morning? ____________
   What time did you get out of bed? ________________
6. Approximately how many hours did you sleep last night? ______
   ____
7. How many hours did you allot for sleep last night (time elapsed from "lights out" to "out of bed")? ________________
8. Rate the quality of last night's sleep:

1	2	3	4	5
excellent				poor

9. Sleep medications taken ________________

night, you may feel more anxious about your sleep. That's why you need only estimate within thirty minutes the time it took you to fall asleep or the length of a nighttime awakening.

After you have completed the 60-Second Sleep Diary for seven consecutive mornings, you are ready to determine your baseline sleep pattern. Using your seven sleep diaries, answer the following questions:

- How many nights per week do you have difficulty falling asleep? ______ On these nights, how much time, on average, does it take you to fall asleep? ______
- How many nights per week do you wake up and have difficulty falling back to sleep? ______ On these nights, how often do you typically wake up? ______ On average, what is the total amount of time that you lie awake during the night after these awakenings? ______
- How many days per week is your final wake-up earlier than desired? ______
- On nights when you have insomnia, how many hours on average do you sleep? ______
- On nights when you don't have insomnia, how many hours on average do you sleep? ______
- How many nights per week do you experience a good night of sleep? ______
- How many nights per week do you take sleeping pills? ______ On these nights, what is the average number of pills you take? ______ What is the typical dose? ______
- What is your average sleep-quality rating on a scale of 1 to 5? ______

Your answers to these questions represent your baseline sleep pattern, which will serve as an objective reference point that will allow you to monitor the improvements in your sleep during this program. Therefore, it is important to keep a record of your baseline sleep pattern for future reference. There is another benefit to objectively assessing your baseline sleep pattern: you may realize that you are actually sleeping better than you think!

Once you have established your baseline, you should continue to fill out the 60-Second Sleep Diary each morning throughout the six-week program described in the following chapters. Completing the diary throughout this program is essential for tracking improvements in your sleep and aiding you in using many of the techniques described subsequently.

Assessing the Thoughts and Behaviors That Are Disrupting Your Sleep

Once you have established your baseline sleep pattern, you are ready to assess the factors that are disturbing your sleep. Let's begin by assessing your sleep-scheduling behaviors.

Your Sleep-Scheduling Behaviors

Your sleep-scheduling behaviors include when you go to bed, how much time you spend in bed, when you get out of bed, and whether you nap. In an effort to cope with insomnia, many insomniacs, such as Jonathan, engage in multiple sleep-scheduling behaviors that disturb sleep.

Jonathan believed that the best way to compensate for insomnia was to go to bed early and to sleep later on weekends in an effort to catch up on the sleep he lost during the week. And even though Jonathan averaged only five hours of sleep per night, he routinely spent eight hours in bed each night. Because Jonathan worked at home two days a week, he also took long afternoon naps in an effort to catch up on his sleep.

Although these strategies may have helped Jonathan to cope with insomnia in the short term, he didn't realize that, in the long run, these sleep-scheduling behaviors were actually exacerbating his insomnia by altering his body-temperature rhythm and weakening his brain's sleep system.

• • •

To assess your sleep-scheduling behaviors, answer the following questions using your sleep diaries as a reference.

- What time do you usually get into bed? _____ Get out of bed? ____
- Does the amount of time that you spend in bed exceed the amount of time that you actually sleep? _____ If so, by how much? ________________________________
- Do you have an inconsistent rising time or sleep later on weekends compared to weekdays? ________________________
- Do you nap? _____ If yes, how many times per week and for how long? ____

Later, we'll explore in detail how these maladaptive sleep-scheduling behaviors cause insomnia and how to improve your sleep by changing these behaviors.

Is Your Bedroom a Learned Cue for Wakefulness?

Mary did all of her television viewing in her bedroom. She also graded her students' papers and spent a lot of time talking on her telephone while lying on her bed. During the hour prior to bedtime, Mary and her husband often discussed emotionally charged topics. When she couldn't sleep, Mary simply stayed in bed in the belief that if she simply tried harder, sleep would eventually come.

Contrary to what many insomniacs think, these behaviors do not aid sleep. Rather, they disturb sleep and heighten insomnia by causing bedtime, the bedroom, and the bed to become learned cues for wakefulness rather than relaxation, drowsiness, and sleep. Assess whether you are engaging in similar behaviors that are contributing to insomnia:

- Do you use your bedroom as an office, for watching television, or for talking on the telephone? ______
- Do you go to bed when your spouse/significant other does or because the 10:00 or 11:00 P.M. news is over rather than because you are drowsy? ______
- Do you toss and turn and try to force sleep when you can't fall asleep? ______
- Do you fall asleep easily anywhere except your bedroom? ______
- Do you work on the computer, pay bills, or discuss problems or emotional issues with your spouse/significant other during the hour before bedtime? ______

Later, we will explore proven techniques for improving sleep by changing these sleep-incompatible behaviors.

How Do You Think About Your Sleep?

Next, assess whether the way you think about your sleep is exacerbating your insomnia.

- Are you anxious about insomnia or perhaps do you fear it?
- Do you tell yourself you won't be able to function during the day if you don't sleep well?
- Do you tell yourself you must have eight hours' sleep to perform effectively?
- Do you always blame poor daytime functioning on insomnia?

As we will soon explore, negative stressful thoughts about sleep only serve to exacerbate insomnia. You'll learn how to recognize and challenge these distorted, negative thoughts and replace them with more positive, accurate thoughts about sleep. These positive thoughts will relax you and improve your sleep.

Lifestyle Behaviors and Your Sleep Environment

In this section, you will assess lifestyle behaviors that affect your sleep and determine whether your sleep environment is conducive to sleep.

First, do you engage in regular physical activity such as walking, running, or other forms of aerobic exercise? Or do you lead a sedentary lifestyle? Whereas regular exercise and physical activity can improve sleep by causing your body-temperature rhythm to rise and fall during the day, lack of physical activity can contribute to insomnia by causing a flattening of your body-temperature rhythm. Exercise may also contribute to more healthy sleep by improving your mood.

David came to my program because he routinely woke up for two or three hours in the middle of the night. Although he had been thinking about starting an exercise program, it wasn't until he learned that exercise can have a beneficial effect on sleep that he started jogging. Within a week, David noticed that he was sleeping more deeply and was waking for significantly shorter periods of time. Within a month, David's sleep was significantly improved.

We will review the positive effects of exercise on sleep. We will also explore various types of exercise, how to start an exercise program, and the beneficial effects of exercise on mood and health.

Consider another factor: do you receive regular exposure to sunlight? Recall that sunlight is an important timing mechanism for sleep. Light is also important for improving mood and energy. If you work indoors, you may be exacerbating insomnia by restricting your exposure to sunlight. We will soon examine the beneficial effects of light on sleep, mood, and health. We'll also review techniques for strengthening your sleep rhythm by increasing exposure to sunlight or artificial bright light.

How about your use of caffeinated beverages in the late afternoon or early evening? Do you drink more than two caffeinated beverages per day? Caffeine can impair sleep by virtue of its stimulant and withdrawal effects.

Lee often felt wide awake at bedtime and usually took a least an hour to fall asleep. When Lee was asked about his caffeine use, he replied that he routinely drank coffee or cola in the afternoon and ate chocolate before bedtime. Lee did not realize that the caffeine in coffee, cola, and chocolate was probably making it more difficult for him to fall asleep.

Shortly, you will learn about the effects of caffeine-containing beverages, foods, and medications on sleep and how to minimize these effects.

And what about your consumption of alcoholic beverages in the evening? How many do you drink and how often? As we will explore in chapter 7, alcohol may help you fall asleep more easily, but it can diminish deep sleep and cause you to wake up during the night. And if you are abusing alcohol, you may be contributing to long-term impairment of your sleep.

Here are four questions to determine if you are abusing alcohol.

1. Have you ever felt you should cut down on your drinking?
2. Have people annoyed you by criticizing your drinking?
3. Have you ever felt bad or guilty about your drinking?
4. Have you ever had a drink first thing in the morning to steady your nerves or to get rid of a hangover?

If you answered yes to any of these questions, you may be abusing alcohol and should consider seeking professional evaluation and treatment.

Smoking is another lifestyle behavior that can disturb sleep. If you smoke near bedtime or after waking during the night, the stimulant and withdrawal effects of nicotine may keep you awake. Smokers experience more sleep problems than nonsmokers, and smokers who quit smoking usually experience improved sleep. In chapter 7 we will explore the effects of nicotine on sleep and how to minimize these effects.

Finally, assess whether or not your sleep environment is conducive to sleep.

1. Is your sleep routinely disturbed by noises such as those made by family members, neighbors, or traffic?
2. Is the temperature of your bedroom comfortable at night?
3. Is your bedroom dark?
4. Is your bed comfortable? If you sleep with a partner, is your bed large enough?

Excessive noise and light can disturb sleep. So, too, can a bedroom that is too warm or too cold, an uncomfortable bed, and sleeping with a partner in a bed that is too small. In chapter 7 we will explore techniques for creating the ideal sleep environment.

Is Daytime Stress Causing Insomnia?

Andrew had another stressful day. It started with a broken button on his shirt collar. Then, on the way to work, a broken water main caused a traffic jam. After arriving late to work, Andrew received e-mail informing him that he would not be receiving a cost of living raise this year. And when he went to the credit union at lunch, the computers were down and the line was out the door.

When Andrew got home, his kids were fighting and his wife was upset that he had forgotten to pick up the dry cleaning. The grass needed to be cut and the toilet was running again.

By the time Andrew went to bed, his mind was racing and he had a headache. No wonder it took him several hours to fall asleep.

As Andrew's story illustrates, we face a multitude of stressors in our work, family, and personal lives. Although some people cope well with daily stress, others experience negative emotional and physical responses that can disturb sleep, health, and well-being.

Stress and insomnia are inextricably linked: insomnia often begins in response to a stressful life event such as a death or divorce; it is one of the first warning signs of excessive daily stress; and many chronic insomniacs have a harder time sleeping after a stressful day.

To assess your current stress level, complete the following two stress inventories; they are the same ones I use with my patients.

STRESS INVENTORY 1

For each area of daily stress, circle the number that corresponds to your perception of stress with 1 being no stress and 10 being the worst possible stress.

Work	1	2	3	4	5	6	7	8	9	10
Family	1	2	3	4	5	6	7	8	9	10
Social Life	1	2	3	4	5	6	7	8	9	10
Finances	1	2	3	4	5	6	7	8	9	10
Health	1	2	3	4	5	6	7	8	9	10
Living Situation	1	2	3	4	5	6	7	8	9	10
Neighborhood	1	2	3	4	5	6	7	8	9	10

STRESS INVENTORY 2

The following is a checklist of some common stress warning signs. Check those that you experience on a weekly basis.

Feelings of frustration or anger ______
Racing or pounding heart ______

Feelings of agitation _____
Shallow or irregular breathing _____
Feeling on edge _____
Headaches _____
Stiff neck or shoulders _____
Upset stomach, excess gas, indigestion, diarrhea, or constipation _____
Cold or sweaty palms _____
Frequent urination _____

If you circled an 8 or higher on at least two of the scales on Stress Inventory 1 and you checked at least two of the warning signs on Stress Inventory 2, you are probably experiencing high levels of daily stress.

The stress-management techniques described in subsequent chapters will teach you to manage excessive stress by learning to relax your mind and body each day. You will also learn to manage stress by recognizing and changing negative stressful thoughts and by developing stress-reducing attitudes and beliefs. By gaining more control over stress, you'll sleep a lot better and your state of mind and health will also improve.

Medical Problems, Drugs, and Mental Health Problems

One of the central themes of this book is that thoughts and behaviors play the primary role in most cases of chronic insomnia. However, medical and mental health problems, certain underlying sleep disorders, and various drugs can contribute to disturbed sleep or even play a primary role in some cases of chronic insomnia. Therefore, assessing whether these factors are affecting your sleep is an important part of your insomnia self-assessment.

Even if a medical or mental health problem, an underlying sleep disorder, or a drug is playing a role in your chronic insomnia, it is important to keep in mind that your thoughts and behaviors are still playing a primary role in your insomnia. Therefore, the techniques in this book should be used in conjunction with any treatment you receive for medical or mental health problems that may be disturbing your sleep.

Medical Problems That Can Affect Sleep

A wide range of medical problems can disturb sleep. Sometimes, the medical causes of poor sleep are obvious, such as pain from arthritis. At other times, the deleterious effects of medical problems on sleep are not so obvious, as in the case of hyperthyroidism.

The following is a list of some common medical problems that can disturb sleep. If you suspect that you have any of these problems, or if you haven't seen your doctor in a while, schedule a thorough medical evaluation so that he or she can more thoroughly evaluate whether any of these problems may be affecting your sleep.

- Angina, a condition in which the heart receives insufficient oxygen, thereby causing pain that can disturb sleep
- Asthma, bronchitis, and emphysema, conditions that disturb sleep by interfering with breathing
- Allergies, congestion, or coughing
- Indigestion, reflux, or ulcers, which are gastrointestinal conditions that disrupt sleep by causing heartburn or acid regurgitation; these conditions can be treated with dietary changes and medication
- Bladder problems such as frequent urination
- Arthritis and chronic pain conditions
- Headaches
- Epilepsy, which causes abnormal electrical activity in the brain that can disturb sleep
- Hyperthyroidism, a condition caused by an overproductive thyroid gland
- Kidney disease
- Diabetes and hypoglycemia
- Dementia or Alzheimer's disease, both of which can cause nighttime agitation, confusion, and insomnia

Medical Conditions Specific to Women

There are a number of women's medical conditions that can disturb sleep. For example, insomnia is common during the last trimester of pregnancy. This can be caused by the stress of the pregnancy and anticipation of the birth or by fetal movements and the physical discomfort of pregnancy.

Patti, who was eight months pregnant, did not look forward to bedtime. She had a hard time falling asleep, in part because she could not get comfortable and because she often found herself thinking about the stress of labor. Once asleep, Patti woke up repeatedly during the night, either because she felt hot or because of the pressure on her bladder caused by her fetus. By the time Patti woke up in the morning, she felt exhausted. Even though she believed caffeine was not good for her fetus, she often drank a cup of coffee in the morning to get herself going.

Although some insomnia is normal and unavoidable during pregnancy, regular insomnia like Patti's, during the last trimester, can be managed by using the techniques in parts II and III of this book. These techniques can also ensure that short-term insomnia during pregnancy doesn't evolve into chronic insomnia. The stress-management techniques in part III can also be a valuable asset in managing the stress and anxiety that many women (and men!) experience during pregnancy.

Menopause is another medical condition that can disrupt women's sleep. The hormonal changes associated with menopause may be one cause of these sleep difficulties; another is the hot flashes of menopause, which result in sensations of increased body temperature and night sweats that are disruptive to sleep. Many women also experience emotional changes and depression during menopause that can contribute to insomnia.

If you are menopausal, talk with your doctor about the available treatments for menopause, which may lead to improved sleep. You should also practice the techniques in this book to minimize menopause-related sleep disturbances and to prevent shot-term insomnia from becoming chronic. Recent research suggests that the relaxation techniques described in part III can be effective in reducing the frequency and severity of menopausal hot flashes.

Premenstrual syndrome (PMS) is another medical condition that can disrupt sleep. For some women, sleep difficulties coincide with the onset of the menses and the negative mood that can occur at this time. Many of my female patients have found the techniques in this program to be effective for minimizing PMS-related sleep problems.

Prescription and Over-the-Counter Drugs

A significant number of prescription and over-the-counter (OTC) drugs can disturb sleep either by causing stimulant or withdrawal effects. Drugs can also impair the quality of your sleep by suppressing deep sleep or dream sleep.

If you are taking prescription drugs, ask your doctor if the drugs may be disturbing your sleep and whether modifying the medication dose or even switching to another related medication that won't adversely affect your sleep is possible. In some cases, simply taking the medication earlier may eliminate sleep problems. If you are taking an OTC, read the medication label carefully or ask your pharmacist if you are uncertain whether it contains sleep-disrupting ingredients.

Listed below are some common types of prescription and OTC medications that can disturb sleep.

- Analgesics that contain caffeine, such as Anacin and Excedrin
- Prescription diet pills
- Steroids
- Beta blockers and some other drugs used for treating high blood pressure
- Nasal decongestants that contain stimulants
- Asthma medications that have stimulating effects

- Thyroid hormones
- Some antidepressant medications
- Drugs for Parkinson's disease

Illicit Drugs

Illicit drugs such as cocaine and amphetamines (speed) have powerful stimulant effects that can make it harder to fall asleep. These drugs can also compromise sleep quality by reducing deep sleep and dream sleep. Because cocaine and amphetamines are highly addictive, they can also cause withdrawal effects that affect sleep.

Marijuana is a widely used recreational drug that can have variable effects on sleep. For some users, marijuana can have relaxing, sedating properties; for others, it can act as a stimulant and make it harder to fall asleep. Research also suggests that long-term marijuana use can impair sleep by reducing dream sleep.

If you are using illicit drugs, your sleep may improve if you stop. If you can't quit, you should consider seeking professional treatment.

Mental Health Problems

DEPRESSION Everyone feels sad or blue at times. However, about 10 to 20 percent of Americans experience serious depression at some point in their lives, and the numbers are growing. Serious depression, called major depression, can be caused by a variety of factors, including genetics, loneliness, lack of social support, alcohol or drug use, negative life events, and negative thinking.

Insomnia, particularly sleep-maintenance insomnia and early morning awakening, is a hallmark symptom of major depression. Some depressed individuals may instead exhibit excessive sleep, called hypersomnia.

Depressed people exhibit a number of other sleep disturbances, including reduced deep sleep, increased light sleep, and excessive REM sleep. They enter REM sleep earlier in the night and spend a greater percentage of time in REM sleep than nondepressed people. Recent research also suggests that the dream content of depressed people is more depressing than that of nondepressed people.

These findings concerning REM sleep disturbances in depression, coupled with the fact that antidepressant drugs work in part by suppressing REM sleep, suggest that abnormalities in dream sleep may be a cause of major depression. Interestingly, research has demonstrated that REM sleep deprivation (accomplished by waking people whenever they start to dream) can produce the same antidepressant effects as antidepressant medications. Unfortunately, REM sleep deprivation is unpleasant and impractical.

Another physiological abnormality associated with depression is a flattened body-temperature rhythm; that is, a depressed person's body temperature doesn't rise and fall as much during the day as that of a nondepressed person. As you will recall, insomniacs exhibit the same problem with their body-temperature rhythm. This irregular rhythm in depressed people, which may be the result of the increased fatigue and reduced physical activity that accompany depression, may ultimately exacerbate insomnia and depressed mood.

Major depression doesn't just affect sleep, it also affects the way we think, behave, and interact with others. When one is depressed, one feels hopeless, helpless, and experiences little pleasure or joy in life. Depressed people are also at greater risk for a variety of health problems, such as cardiovascular diseases and lowered life expectancy. Depression also weakens our immune systems and is a risk factor for suicide. Therefore, if you are experiencing major depression, it is essential that you seek professional evaluation and treatment.

To help you determine whether you have major depression, think about whether you have experienced any of the following symptoms nearly every day for a two-week period in the past few months.

1. A relatively prominent, persistent depressed mood that is characterized by feeling sad, blue, hopeless, low, down in the dumps, and irritable

2. Loss of interest or pleasure in all or almost all usual activities and pastimes
3. Poor appetite or significant weight loss when not dieting or increased appetite and significant weight gain
4. Insomnia
5. Restlessness or lethargy that is observable by others
6. Loss of interest in sexual activity
7. Fatigue or loss of energy
8. Feelings of worthlessness or guilt
9. Diminished ability to think or concentrate
10. Thoughts of death or suicide

If you have experienced symptom 1 or 2 and at least four of symptoms 3–10, you may have major depression and should seek professional evaluation and treatment.

Major depression can be successfully treated in several ways. One treatment involves the use of antidepressant medications such as Prozac, which are highly effective in about 70 percent of cases. These medications, which are not addicting, usually take a few weeks to lessen depression and may cause some temporary side effects, such as dry mouth and constipation.

The most effective nondrug treatment for depression is cognitive therapy. The word *cognitive* relates to your thoughts. Cognitive therapy is based on the premise that our negative moods and stress come from our negative, distorted thoughts. Cognitive therapy for depression involves learning to recognize, challenge, and change the negative, distorted thinking patterns that cause depressed moods. For many depressed people, cognitive therapy can be as effective as antidepressant medication—without the side effects. In some cases, the most effective treatment for depression involves a combination of cognitive therapy and antidepressant medication.

If you have some but not all of the symptoms of major depression, you have what is called mild or moderate depression. Sometimes, chronic insomnia can be the cause; in these cases, using the techniques in this book to improve sleep will also result in improved mood. As we will explore later, exercise can also be effective in alleviating mild to moderate depression.

ANXIETY Anxiety is another prevalent mental health problem that can disturb sleep. Anxiety is a feeling of apprehension, worry, or fear that differs from stress in a fundamental way. Whereas stress involves a reaction to an identifiable external stressor or event, anxiety occurs in the absence of any identifiable event or precipitator.

Some anxiety is beneficial. It allows us to plan, search for alternatives, rehearse actions, and prepare for negative outcomes. But when we experience too much anxiety, our sleep, work, sense of pleasure, and relationships can suffer.

Excessive, maladaptive anxiety that interferes with daily living is called generalized anxiety disorder (GAD). GAD is characterized by persistent, excessive, unrealistic, uncontrollable worry that causes the person to constantly feel on edge. People with GAD cannot relax and enjoy life; they feel chronically irritable, have a harder time concentrating on things, report more sleep problems, and are at greater risk for numerous health problems such as high blood pressure, abnormal heart rhythms, heart attacks, and sudden death from heart disease.

The physical symptoms of GAD include

- Shakiness, jitteriness, trembling, or jumpiness
- Eyelid twitching, furrowed brow, or strained face
- Heart pounding or racing, sweating, cold and clammy hands, or dry mouth
- A knot in the stomach, a lump in the throat, or a fast breathing rate

The most common treatment for GAD is antianxiety medication, which is helpful in controlling the problem. However, like sleeping pills, these medications can have side effects such as dependence and tolerance. Some people attempt to self-medicate their anxiety by drinking alcohol. However, alcohol actually increases anxiety.

For many people, cognitive behavioral therapy, in which the individual learns to change the thoughts, behaviors, and bodily responses associated with GAD, can be a highly effective nondrug treatment. The self-help techniques described in part III can also be highly effective in controlling anxiety. In fact, research has consistently shown that these techniques can be as effective as, or more effective than, antianxiety medication. Other self-help techniques for managing anxiety include cutting back on caffeine and exercising, which we will explore in chapter 7.

POST-TRAUMATIC STRESS DISORDER (PTSD) A less common mental health problem that can cause insomnia is post-traumatic stress disorder (PTSD). In PTSD, a traumatic event (such as physical or sexual abuse, war, or a natural disaster) is continually reexperienced emotionally. This chronic "reliving" of the trauma results in fear, anxiety, physical stress responses, insomnia, and nightmares. If you have experienced a trauma and think that you may be suffering from PTSD, you should seek help from a mental health professional who specializes in this condition.

Underlying Sleep Disorders

SLEEP APNEA James, a fifty-year-old man, complained of excessive daytime sleepiness. He was also overweight, had high blood pressure, and often awakened in the morning with a headache. James's wife reported that he snored loudly and often woke briefly during the night, making choking or gasping sounds. James denied any knowledge of this behavior; in fact, he believed he was a sound sleeper.

James has a syndrome called sleep apnea, which is more prevalent in older individuals, men, and overweight people. This sleep disorder causes breathing to stop during sleep for anywhere from ten seconds up to several minutes. These pauses in breathing, called apneas, can occur hundreds of times a night and are more likely to occur in certain positions, particularly when sleeping on the back. If apnea is severe enough, the sleeper wakes gasping for breath and may never get more than five minutes of uninterrupted sleep all night.

When apnea occurs, the cessation in breathing causes a drop in blood oxygen levels, forcing the heart to labor harder to keep the blood oxygenated. For this reason, sleep apnea is a risk factor for hypertension, strokes, and heart disease. It can also cause chronic sleep disruption that may leave the patient feeling exhausted and sleepy during the day. In some cases of sleep apnea, daytime sleepiness can be severe enough to cause car accidents. In fact, a recent study found that people who have sleep apnea are seven times more likely to get into a car accident than the rest of the population. Therefore, if you experience symptoms while you sleep such as loud snoring interrupted by periods of silence for ten seconds or longer, feeling unable to breath, or making gasping sounds, you may have sleep apnea and should be evaluated at a sleep disorders center.

There are multiple causes of apnea. These include a problem in the brain's respiration center; obstruction of the breathing passages caused by the tongue, tonsils or adenoids, fat deposits, or excess tissue in the throat; and structural abnormalities in the throat or jaw. The self-help treatments for apnea include avoiding sleeping on your back (by wearing a T-shirt to bed that has a tennis ball sewn into the back of it, you will be less likely to sleep on your back), using pillows to keep the head elevated, abstaining from alcohol and sleeping pills (which exacerbate sleep apnea), and losing weight.

The most effective medical treatment for sleep apnea is Continuous Positive Airway Pressure (CPAP), in which the person wears in bed a nasal mask that is attached to a machine that pushes air through the nose to keep the breathing passages open. In severe cases of apnea, surgery may be necessary to increase the size of the breathing passages or to correct structural abnormalities in the upper airway.

PERIODIC LIMB MOVEMENTS (PLM) PLM is another disorder that can disturb sleep. PLMs are not the same as the occasional body jerks, called hypnic jerks, that some people experience at the onset of sleep. Rather, PLMs are episodes lasting from a few minutes to several hours during sleep that involve the legs or arms twitching, jerking, or even kicking repeatedly. Like sleep apnea, the interruptions in sleep caused by PLM can leave the person feeling exhausted and sleepy during the day. If you wake up with your bedcovers in disarray, or if a bed partner has told you that you jerk or kick during sleep, you may have PLM and should be evaluated at a sleep disorders center.

Sleep researchers don't really know what causes PLM. Warm baths before bedtime are sometimes helpful in alleviating PLM symptoms. However, muscle-relaxing medications are the most effective treatment. These medications suppress the PLMs or help the person sleep through them, but the medications don't cure PLM and can become addicting. Unfortunately, no satisfactory nondrug treatment for PLM currently exists.

DIAGNOSING SLEEP APNEA AND PLM USING ALL-NIGHT SLEEP STUDIES Sleep apnea and PLM can be definitively diagnosed only by an all-night sleep study. These studies are conducted at a sleep disorders clinic, which has private rooms that resemble a bedroom or hotel room complete with bathroom, television, and radio. On the night of the study, the patient arrives an hour before his or her usual bedtime and is hooked up for the sleep recording. This procedure involves attaching several electrodes to the scalp to create an electroencephalogram (EEG), which measures brain waves, and to the chin and around the eyes to measure muscle tension and eye movements. Sensors are also placed on the body to measure blood oxygen levels (this is usually done by attaching a meter to the earlobe), respiration, heart rate, and leg movements. An all-night sleep study is called a polysomnogram, because multiple physiological measures are recorded while the individual is asleep.

Once the patient is hooked up, he or she is asked to go to sleep while the multiple physiological measurements are obtained throughout the night. In the morning, the polysomnogram is analyzed by a sleep specialist, who can determine whether the patient actually suffers from sleep apnea or PLM.

RESTLESS LEGS Restless legs is a disorder that causes unpleasant sensations in the legs while lying down. These sensations, which are often described as a creeping or crawling sensation in the calves, typically occur at bedtime when the person is still awake, and can therefore make it difficult to fall asleep. Many people with PLM also have restless legs syndrome, and almost all people with restless legs have PLM.

The sensations by restless legs result in a strong urge to move the legs, massage them, or walk around, all of which alleviate the discomfort. Self-help techniques for this disorder include exercise, elimination of caffeine, and some dietary supplements such as iron, calcium, and folic acid. The usual medical treatment for restless legs involves various types of sedative medications that can reduce the severity of this condition but can't cure it.

DELAYED PHASE DISORDER Individuals with this disorder can't fall asleep until late at night, often around 3:00 or 4:00 A.M. Once asleep, however, they usually sleep well for seven or eight hours and awaken feeling refreshed.

The opposite of delayed phase disorder is advanced phase disorder. This condition, which is most common among the elderly, is characterized by falling asleep early in the evening, around 8:00 P.M. for example, then waking in the predawn hours and being unable to fall back to sleep.

Delayed and advanced phase disorders are caused by a body-temperature rhythm that either falls too late or too early at night, respectively. These disorders are treated at sleep disorders centers by using artificial bright-light boxes to normalize the body-temperature rhythm.

NIGHTMARES A nightmare is a frightening dream that usually involves themes of danger, being chased, being killed, or falling. Because our muscles are paralyzed when we dream, we feel trapped during a nightmare and therefore wake up feeling fearful and agitated. Nightmares usually occur in the second half of the night, when dream sleep is more prominent.

Although occasional nightmares are normal, frequent nightmares are not. They are caused by a number of factors, including traumatic events such as abuse or natural disasters, or by underlying psychological conflicts that have not been adequately resolved.

One treatment for nightmares is the use of psychotherapy to alleviate the underlying conflict causing them. Another treatment involves behavioral therapy in which the nightmare sufferer is trained to write down the content of the nightmare, rewrite it with a different outcome, and to mentally rehearse this new outcome daily.

BRUXISM (TOOTH GRINDING) If you grind your teeth while you sleep, you may have bruxism. This disorder can result in tooth damage and morning jaw pain or headaches. The most common treatment is a rubber mouth guard that is worn to bed to prevent the grinding. However, bruxism also seems to be exacerbated by stress. Many patients who practice the stress-reduction techniques in part III of this book report significant improvement in symptoms of bruxism.

The Next Step

You have now completed your insomnia self-assessment. You should have a greater understanding of the particular thoughts and behaviors that are causing your insomnia. Now you are ready to begin the six-week program presented in chapters 5 through 10, in which you will learn more about why these thoughts and behaviors cause insomnia and, most important, step-by-step techniques for changing them.

You will begin this program by learning one of its most powerful techniques: cognitive restructuring. This technique will teach you how to improve your sleep by changing the way you think about your sleep. It will also be the initial catalyst for improving yourself and your life in a number of important ways.

PART II

CHANGING SLEEP THOUGHTS AND BEHAVIORS

CHAPTER FIVE

Changing Your Thoughts About Sleep

Lauren, a thirty-five-year-old freelance writer, can still recall lying awake at night as a child. By the time she graduated from college, Lauren's life had become a never-ending focus on insomnia. She couldn't go to bed or wake up during the night without panicking about whether she would fall asleep, and she worried constantly about how she would function during the day and whether her insomnia would cause a serious health problem. As evening approached, Lauren became increasingly apprehensive about whether she would have to face another night of insomnia so that, by bedtime, she feared turning out the lights. She couldn't imagine what it was like not to worry about sleep and could only wonder whether she would ever sleep more than five hours a night again.

Lauren's experience probably sounds very familiar. That's because her stressful preoccupation with sleep is shared by most insomniacs. Of all the factors that cause insomnia, this consuming, negative thinking about sleep plays the most salient role. Even if you realize that this negative thinking aggravates your insomnia, you probably feel powerless to do anything about it, which makes the problem of insomnia even more frustrating and exasperating.

Think about what this means. If your thinking can cause insomnia, can't it also overcome insomnia? As you will learn in this chapter, it can! In fact, changing your negative thoughts about sleep—called cognitive restructuring—is one of the most powerful techniques you will learn in this book. The use of this technique will have a profound beneficial effect on your sleep and will also provide these other important benefits:

- You will begin to understand the powerful effect your thoughts have on your emotions and body; you will also learn to control negative thoughts and emotions and think more positively.
- You will boost your confidence and sense of control over sleep because you will see that the power to conquer insomnia resides within you and your thoughts.
- You will set the stage for the cognitive stress-management techniques that you will learn later in this program.

In short, cognitive restructuring will be the initial catalyst for improving your sleep and yourself in a number of important ways.

Let's begin by examining some recent scientific findings concerning the placebo effect and the new field of psychoneuroimmunology. These exciting findings, which have precipitated a change in the way science looks at the mind and the body, will help you to understand the powerful effect your thoughts about sleep have on your insomnia. They will also help you realize that your thoughts have a greater effect on your emotions and body than you ever realized.

The Placebo Effect and Psychoneuroimmunology

You may be surprised to learn that, prior to the 1900s, most medicines given by physicians were worthless. Yet, remarkably, patients still improved. How was this possible? It was due to the patient's *belief* in the physician and the medicine, which mobilized strong self-healing mechanisms. This is called the placebo effect and it is recognized as a powerful component of all medical treatments.

In a dramatic case study done on the placebo effect during the 1950s, a woman who suffered nausea and vomiting during pregnancy was given a medication by her doctor and told that the medication was "new" and "effective" and that it would quickly relieve her symptoms. Within twenty minutes, the woman's nausea and vomiting stopped even though she in fact had taken ipecac, a medication that induces vomiting! This study demonstrated that the woman's belief in the drug was so strong, it counteracted the physiological action of the drug.

Today, newly developed medications are scientifically evaluated by being compared to an inactive placebo pill. Study after study has shown that, for virtually all health problems, including anxiety, depression, pain, fever, headaches, seasickness, high blood pressure, angina, acne, asthma, insomnia, ulcers, and arthritis, about one-third of patients improve when given a placebo. In fact, about one-third of patients in pain will respond as well to a placebo as they will to morphine, which is the most powerful narcotic ever developed! If a new medication were discovered that had the same powerful healing properties as the placebo effect, it would undoubtedly be hailed as a miracle drug.

If you take sleeping pills, you probably do not realize that you have already experienced the placebo effect. Recall that sleeping pills lose their effectiveness after six weeks of regular use. Therefore, if you have been taking sleeping pills for more than a few months and they still put you to sleep, it's the placebo effect working, not the pill. Likewise, if over-the-counter sleep aids are no more effective than a sugar pill, why do they seem to work for many insomniacs? Because the placebo effect is at work! And if you fall asleep in less than twenty minutes after taking a sleeping pill, it's the placebo effect in action—no sleeping pill works that fast!

Although we don't know the exact mechanism underlying the placebo effect, it is probably due to the effects our thoughts have on our brain and body chemistry. However it works, the placebo effect is one of the best pieces of scientific evidence demonstrating that thoughts can have significant effects on our moods and bodies. The very power of the placebo effect means that, by maximizing your belief in the techniques in this program, your sleep will improve as it did for Robin.

When Robin first contacted me by telephone to inquire about my insomnia program, I described the program and its success in helping patients to conquer insomnia. By the time Robin and I met for her initial appointment, her sleep had already improved significantly. Why? Because her *belief* that the program was going to work for her created a placebo effect that produced beneficial changes in her emotions, body, and sleep.

Recent scientific research on the relationship between the mind and the immune system has given rise to the field of psyhoneuroimmunology (PNI). PNI research, which exemplifies some of the most rigorous research in mind-body medicine, has challenged the traditional separation of the mind and the immune system by demonstrating that mental stress of various kinds, including loneliness, bereavement, marital separation, and divorce, decreases immune functioning. For example, a PNI study published in the *New England Journal of Medicine* demonstrated that individuals with higher levels of psychological stress were at greater risk for developing the common cold. PNI research has also demonstrated that relaxation techniques can strengthen the functioning of the immune system.

Negative Sleep Thoughts

Just as the placebo effect and PNI demonstrate that our thoughts can affect our emotions and our bodies, negative sleep thoughts (NSTs) can have a profound adverse effect on sleep. Below are some examples of NSTs, which will likely sound very familiar:

> **"I didn't sleep a wink last night."**
> **"I must get eight hours of sleep."**
> **"My insomnia is going to cause health problems."**

"I'm dreading bedtime."
"Why does sleep come so easily for everyone but me?"
"I feel miserable because I didn't sleep well."
"How will I function today after such a horrible night of sleep?"
"I can't sleep without a sleeping pill."

How do you think these NSTs affect your sleep? The answer is simple. When they occur at bedtime or while you are awake in the middle of the night, NSTs have a forceful effect on making you feel anxious and frustrated. In turn, these negative emotions mobilize the stress response, which increases your heart rate, blood pressure, muscle tension, and breathing rate and speeds up your brain waves. (I will discuss the stress response in detail in chapter 8.) The stress response then activates your brain's wakefulness system and weakens the sleep system. You can guess the result—another night of insomnia.

NSTs share a number of important features. One is that they occur almost automatically, like a knee-jerk reaction, so that you are not always aware of them or their negative impact on your sleep. Another, as you will explore in this chapter, is that NSTs are often inaccurate and distorted, especially when they occur in the quiet and darkness of the night. Also, NSTs often seem like normal, appropriate reactions to insomnia. However, the only purpose they serve is to make it more difficult to fall asleep.

Cognitive Restructuring

Now that you understand NSTs and their harmful effect on your sleep, the next step is to learn to change your NSTs using cognitive restructuring. (*Cognitive restructuring* means to change your thoughts.)

The aim of cognitive restructuring is simple yet powerful: by recognizing and replacing your NSTs with more accurate, positive thoughts about sleep you will be less anxious and frustrated about insomnia. As a result, you will relax and sleep better. *Keep in mind, however, that this is not the same as denying insomnia. Rather, cognitive restructuring means to think about insomnia in less negative and distorted ways.*

Before you can use cognitive restructuring to improve your sleep, you must first learn about some important scientific findings concerning sleep and insomnia.

The Eight-Hour-Sleep Myth

Do you tell yourself that if you don't get eight hours of sleep, you won't be able to function during the day? Many insomniacs such as Jody do. When she first came to my program, Jody told me she needed "at least eight hours of sleep a night to function effectively, and the more sleep I get, the better." Another patient of mine who frequently traveled for business would often tell her husband, "Because I've got a very early flight tomorrow I'm going to get less than seven hours of sleep tonight, which means I'm going to feel miserable tomorrow."

However, the belief that everyone must get eight hours of sleep is a myth. People are not the same height and weight and their sleep needs vary as well Although adults average just under seven and a half hours of nighttime sleep, many individuals function effectively on less. In fact, about 20 percent of the population sleeps six or fewer hours per night, and research shows that some adults function well with as little as three hours per night. There is even some research to suggest that too much sleep can cause us to feel lethargic.

Here are three questions to determine whether you are getting enough sleep:

1. Do you need an alarm clock to wake up?
2. Do you habitually sleep late on weekends?
3. Do you frequently fall asleep during meetings, lectures, boring or sedentary activities, or while watching television?

If you answered no to each of these questions, you may be getting enough sleep and trying to get more sleep than you really need.

The message here is fundamental: try to modify unrealistic beliefs that you may hold about your sleep requirements. NSTs such as "I can't function with less than eight hours of sleep" may not be accurate and will make you more anxious and more likely to experience insomnia. By believing that you can function with less than eight hours of sleep, you will control NSTs and fall asleep more easily.

You Are Getting More Sleep Than You Think

If I asked you how much sleep you obtained last night, how accurate do you think your answer would be? Do you think thoughts such as "I didn't sleep a wink last night" or "I haven't slept in days" are realistic?

Studies consistently show that insomniacs are not accurate in estimating how much sleep they obtain. This is because they overestimate the time it takes to fall asleep and their time awake during the night; they also underestimate total sleep time compared to objective brain-wave sleep recordings.

Hard to believe? In a study at the Stanford University Sleep Clinic, 122 insomniacs spent the night in a sleep lab so that their sleep could be measured with brain-wave recordings. On the average, these individuals overestimated the time it took them to fall asleep by thirty minutes and underestimated total sleep time by one hour.

Why do insomniacs exhibit this sleep "misperception"? One reason is that they incorrectly perceive light stages of sleep, such as Stage 2 sleep, as wakefulness. However, recall that Stage 2 sleep is a bona fide sleep stage as illustrated by the fact that adults spend half the night and the elderly spend most of the night in this stage. Use this knowledge on nights when you slept lightly and weren't sure if you were awake or sleep—it is very likely you were in Stage 2 sleep!

The other reason insomniacs exhibit this sleep misperception is that, in unpleasant circumstances such as lying awake in bed from insomnia, the subjective perception of time is longer than actual clock time. Conversely, in relaxing and pleasant situations, we underestimate duration of elapsed time. If you take a moment, I'm sure you can recall unpleasant experiences in which something seemed to "take forever" compared to pleasurable ones in which time seemed to "fly." This is what Albert Einstein meant when he said, "If you are sitting on a hot stove a minute seems like an hour, but if you are doing something pleasurable an hour can seem like a minute." Therefore, if you experience a night when you weren't sure if you were really sleeping but time seemed to pass quickly, you were probably asleep.

Telling yourself that you may be getting more sleep than you think is an effective strategy for overcoming NSTs and improving your sleep.

The Effects of Sleep Loss

What is your greatest worry about insomnia? If you are like most poor sleepers, it's the adverse effects of insomnia on your daytime functioning. This concern is the result of a number of popular misconceptions about the effects of sleep loss, due in part to media reports that are often one-sided and inaccurate. These reports, which emphasize the deleterious effects of sleep loss, are based on the findings of some sleep researchers who believe that most Americans are sleep deprived, are accumulating a dangerous "sleep debt," and need at least eight hours of sleep per night.

However, the media usually fail to present the other side of the story. First of all, there is no consistent scientific evidence that insomnia causes significant health problems, and no one has ever died from insomnia. Also, our daytime functioning is affected by many factors, including stress, nutrition, exercise, alcohol, medication, sunlight, the time of year, and heredity. It is very common for insomniacs, however, to mistakenly attribute their daytime functioning entirely to their lack of sleep. For example, one of my patients stated that her cold was caused by her insomnia. Although it is possible that insomnia increased her susceptibility to catching a cold, it is just as likely that poor nutrition, physical inactivity, stress, or other factors were involved.

Learning not to blame insomnia for all your misfortunes will minimize NSTs and help you relax. Your sleep will improve, as will your confidence in your ability to control your sleep!

Many sleep researchers believe, based on substantial scientific evidence, that we have a remarkable tolerance for sleep loss, at least on a temporary basis. For example, a large number of studies have failed to find significant adverse effects on daytime performance after a poor night's sleep. Even one night of total sleep loss makes healthy young volunteers sleepy, but has no major effect on daytime performance. It is only performance of monotonous or sedentary tasks such as driving, or the ability to produce creative solutions to problems, that seem to deteriorate after one sleepless night.

Even extended sleeplessness may have little effect on us other than making us feel very sleepy. This is illustrated by the case of Randy Gardner, who stayed awake in an experiment for eleven days and established the world record for sleeplessness. Randy did experience increased irritability and drowsiness, but never delusions or hallucinations. When he finally went to bed, he slept for under fifteen hours and afterward felt fine with no ill effects.

By demonstrating that extreme sleep loss does not invariably produce serious consequences, Randy's case can help you to manage NSTs. His case also underscores two facts: we don't need to recover all of the sleep we lose; and if you think you haven't slept in weeks, you are either engaging in very unrealistic NSTs or you have set a new world record!

What about the effects of chronic sleep loss on daytime performance? There is considerable evidence suggesting that, for most individuals, performance on alertness, memory, and problem-solving tasks can be maintained for extended periods of time with about 70 percent of normal sleep, or about five and a half hours for an eight-hour sleeper. Let's examine some of this research.

Sailors, Doctors, and College Students

Some of the most useful findings for challenging NSTs come from studies on sleep in solo transatlantic yacht racers. To win, they try to sleep as little as possible (since they can't maintain course and monitor conditions as effectively when they are asleep) yet obtain enough sleep to maintain performance under the challenging conditions of severe storms, darkness, being lost, or being at risk of collision with large ships. These studies show that the sailors who perform best in these races average five and a half hours of sleep during voyages that last several months.

Studies on college students and physicians also suggest that performance can be maintained with about 70 percent of normal sleep. In one study, for example, long-term gradual sleep loss was studied in adult collegiate couples whose sleep was reduced to five and a half hours per night over an eight-month period. In another study, students were restricted to five and a half hours of sleep for two months. In both studies, there were no significant detrimental effects on cognitive, behavioral, or physiological functioning, suggesting that chronic sleep loss of two to three hours per night for up to eight months does not result in significant consequences.

Physicians undergoing residency training must perform the demands of medicine, including surgery and emergency-room care, for months at a time on restricted sleep. As part of their medical training, residents are required to work ninety- or even one-hundred-hour weeks. Every three or four days, they spend thirty-six hours on call in the hospital responding to emergencies.

During this thirty-six-hour period, residents rarely sleep. Furthermore, even if they slept eight hours a night on each of the five nights a week that they were not on call, residents would still average only about five and a half hours of sleep per night. Neurosurgeons are often on call every other night during their residency training, resulting in even less sleep, yet they are able to handle the demands of brain surgery.

Finally, two other findings about sleep loss will help you diminish NSTs and sleep better. First, studies on insomniacs indicate that they average about five and a half hours of sleep—only two hours fewer than normal sleepers—and do not exhibit poorer daytime performance compared to good sleepers. Second, daytime alertness does not suffer significantly unless sleep is reduced below five and a half hours. These studies suggest that insomnia usually won't impair your daytime alertness or performance.

Core Sleep

It's clear from the research we have explored that your daytime performance will usually not suffer significantly if you obtain about five and a half hours of sleep, or what some sleep researchers call *core sleep*. But why does core sleep maintain performance? Probably because it contains 100 percent of our deep sleep, which, as you will recall, is the most important stage of sleep for daytime functioning.

Many of my patients ask me whether core sleep must be uninterrupted. Recent research suggests that is not the case. Many parents, for example, regularly experience interrupted sleep due to a baby or young child waking during the night, yet still perform effectively during the day. In fact, research on soldiers, fire fighters, and astronauts, who sometimes have to perform on drastically reduced, interrupted sleep, suggests that, by breaking up sleep, a person can function on less time than full core sleep—as little as three hours—without significant consequences.

The Apollo 13 astronauts, for example, were able to guide their disabled spacecraft back to earth while getting about three hours of interrupted sleep for each of four days. Though irritable and exhausted, they functioned under extremely challenging circumstances without any errors. Other studies have shown that people who are allotted thirty-minute naps every four hours, or a total of three hours of sleep during a twenty-four-hour period, can maintain performance.

Another important finding about core sleep: if you don't obtain it one night, your brain will do everything possible to get it the next. How do we know this? Because on nights after sleep loss, the brain compensates by producing an increased percentage of deep sleep and dream sleep, which also explains why we don't have to recover all of the sleep we lose. You can rest assured that your brain is programmed to obtain core sleep.

Sleep is similar to food in that our body also needs a core amount of food to function. Most individuals, however, eat more than their core food requirements to *feel* good. Similarly, we can maintain performance with core sleep for extended periods of time, but most people don't feel their best unless they obtain additional sleep, or what some sleep researchers call *optional* sleep.

In this sense, the impact of losing part or all of a night's sleep is similar to that of skipping a meal or fasting for a day. And just as it is possible to go without food for several days without serious consequences, we can endure a few days without sleep. Yet missing sleep creates anxiety that missing food does not!

Telling yourself that you can function on core sleep is a highly effective strategy for managing NSTs. In fact, this technique has helped almost all of my patients to become more relaxed about sleep and, as a consequence, to sleep better. This strategy will also create a placebo effect that will improve your sleep and your daytime functioning and will empower you with the realization that the ability to control insomnia resides within your thoughts.

Insomnia and Daytime Mood

Since insomnia doesn't have significant effects on daytime alertness or performance, what are its main consequences? Think about this and you will realize that the primary effect of insomnia is impaired daytime mood in the form of irritability, frustration, anxiety, mild depression, fatigue, or reduced motivation. *This realization is important for reducing your fear of insomnia and minimizing NSTs: it means that, in most cases, the worst thing that will happen if you don't sleep well is that your mood may suffer.*

It is also important for you to recognize that, although the daytime mood effects of insomnia are due to sleep loss, they are also the direct result of your NSTs. For example, when you get out of bed in the morning, do you tell yourself, "I slept only five hours, so I'll never be able to function today"? If so, how do you think these

NSTs affect your daytime mood? By creating a negative placebo effect! Because a positive placebo effect can improve your mood, a negative placebo effect can certainly impair it. If you begin your day by thinking that you will have a lousy one, what are the odds you will have a good day?

You can prove to yourself that the daytime mood effects of insomnia are due in part to your NSTs. Recall times in your life when you experienced sleep loss due to pleasurable circumstances such as vacations, late-night socializing or parties, or lovemaking. In contrast to the frustration and aggravation of insomnia, sleep loss under these circumstances does not usually result in impaired daytime mood because these circumstances are under our control and therefore don't give rise to NSTs.

So remember that it's not just sleep loss that hinders your daytime functioning; it's also your NSTs in response to sleep loss. This means that, if you don't sleep well, you can still minimize impaired daytime mood by minimizing your NSTs. This is also a powerful way of using your thoughts to gain greater control over your emotions and daytime functioning.

Using Cognitive Restructuring Every Day

Now that you have explored some important scientific findings concerning sleep and insomnia, you should already be thinking in a more positive and accurate way about your sleep and may already be experiencing improved sleep as a result.

However, to maximize improvement in your sleep, you must learn to consistently recognize and replace your NSTs with more accurate positive thoughts about sleep. This first involves becoming more aware of your NSTs, which is not always easy since NSTs tend to be automatic. That's why you will need to write down your NSTs, which will also help you to see how distorted and inaccurate they are.

Take a moment to look at your 60-Second Sleep Diary at the end of this chapter, which you used to establish your baseline sleep pattern and which you should still be completing each morning. Notice that the diary at the end of this chapter contains a new item for recording NSTs.

When you fill out your 60-Second Sleep Diary each morning, write down any NSTs that you experienced at bedtime, while awake during the night, or upon rising from bed in the morning, and then examine your NSTs. Are they inaccurate? Are they overly negative? Do you use words such as *horrible*, *awful*, or *terrible* to describe a bad night of sleep? The words you use reflect how you think about your sleep.

The next step is to replace your NSTs with more accurate and positive thoughts about sleep, or what I call positive sleep thoughts (PSTs). To make this easier, a list of sample PSTs is provided for you at the end of this chapter. These PSTs are based on the sleep and insomnia research we have explored in this chapter and on the information from chapter 2 on the physiology of sleep. They are the same PSTs my patients use to change NSTs.

Review these PSTs and choose those that appeal most to you, or create your own. Then, each morning, record a PST on your sleep diary below the space for NSTs; this will help you to start thinking PSTs instead of NSTs. Some of my patients even keep this list of PSTs by their beds so that they can read it if they are having trouble sleeping. You may decide to do the same.

To help you systematically track your use of cognitive restructuring, your Week One Progress Summary is also included at the end of this chapter. Take a moment to review the progress summary, which you should complete after reviewing your seven sleep diaries for this week. As you will see, the progress summary contains items that will help you track your current sleep pattern and your use of cognitive restructuring techniques. The summary also contains an item concerning sleeping-pill use. This item will help you track changes in sleep-medication use as you implement the medication-reduction techniques you learned in chapter 3.

If your progress summary indicates that you recorded a PST every day and you are mentally practicing cognitive restructuring regularly, congratulate yourself! If not, you need to make a greater commitment to practicing cognitive restructuring on a daily basis.

As with the 60-Second Sleep Diary, you will continue to complete a weekly progress summary to track improvements in your sleep during the remaining five weeks of this program. In fact, you can objectively determine whether you are already sleeping better by comparing your sleep pattern from the Week One Progress Summary to your baseline sleep pattern from the self-assessment you conducted in chapter 4. You may find that you are already experiencing fewer insomnia nights or using less sleep medication!

Lauren, whom you met at the beginning of this chapter, learned to use this systematic approach to cognitive restructuring to significantly improve her sleep. She did this by first recording her NSTs on her daily sleep diary. These included:

"I don't think I can fall back to sleep."
"I can't fall asleep without a sleeping pill."
"This is going to be another night of insomnia."
"My insomnia is getting worse."
"I need more sleep."
"Oh no, I'm awake!"

Lauren then recorded one of these PSTs each day on her daily sleep diary:

"I always fall back to sleep sooner or later."
"I need less sleep than I thought."
"My sleep is getting better and better."
"My sleep will be improving as I learn these techniques."
"If I get my core sleep, I'll be able to function during the day."

Lauren's results? After one week of practicing cognitive restructuring, Lauren said, "I had the best week of sleep I've had in years." After four weeks, she was sleeping close to seven hours, and after eight weeks, she told me, "I'm amazed to see the progress I've made. I fall asleep easily and quickly and I rarely wake up. I'm sleeping eight hours per night, my energy level is great, and I've learned to think about my sleep without panicking. I have a new sense of confidence and a new view of myself—I'm thrilled!"

By practicing cognitive restructuring each day, you, too, will start to think more positively and confidently about sleep; you'll gain more control over sleep and will soon start to sleep better as a result. You will also see that you can control negative thoughts, think more positively, and realize the powerful beneficial effect your thoughts can have on your emotions, health, and well-being. We'll return to this empowering idea in part III.

60-SECOND SLEEP DIARY

Night ________________ Date ________________

1. Last night, what time did you get into bed? ________________
   Turn the lights off? ____________________________
2. About how long did it take you to fall asleep? ______________
   ____
3. About how many times did you awaken during the night? _____
   ____
4. For each awakening, about how long were you awake? ________
   1st ____________________ 2nd ______________________
   3rd ____________________ 4th ______________________
5. What time was your final wake-up this morning? ___________
   What time did you get out of bed? ___________________
6. Approximately how many hours did you sleep last night? ______
   ____
7. How many hours did you allot for sleep last night (time elapsed from "lights out" to "out of bed")? ___________________
8. Rate the quality of last night's sleep:

1	2	3	4	5
excellent				poor

9. Sleep medications taken ______________________________
10. a) NSTs ____
    b) PSTs ____

POSITIVE SLEEP THOUGHTS

My performance will not suffer significantly if I get my core sleep.

I'm probably getting more sleep than I think.

My daytime functioning is not affected only by my sleep.

Since I have survived nights of insomnia before, I can do it again.

If I didn't sleep well last night, I am more likely to sleep well tonight due to a biological pressure to recover my core sleep.

My daytime malfunctioning is due in part to my NSTs.

Sleep requirements vary from person to person.

There is no evidence that insomnia causes health problems.

In most cases, the worst thing that may happen if I don't sleep well is that my mood will be impaired during the day.

If I awaken after about five and a half hours of sleep, I have gotten my core sleep.

I'm more likely to fall asleep as my body temperature falls throughout the night.

It is normal to initially feel alert if I awaken at the beginning or end of a dream; drowsiness will soon follow.

My functioning will improve during the day as my body temperature rises.

My sleep will be improving as I learn these behavioral techniques.

These techniques have worked for others, and they will work for me.

WEEK ONE PROGRESS SUMMARY

1. Assess your sleep pattern this week by noting:

a) the number of good nights of sleep ______________________

b) the number of nights of core sleep (five and a half hours or more) ______________________

c) the number of insomnia nights ______________________

2. On how many daily sleep diaries did you record a positive sleep thought? ______________________

3. How often did you mentally practice cognitive restructuring this week (circle one)?

this week
regularly
occasionally
never

4. Assess your sleep-medication use this week by noting:

a) the number of medication-free nights ______________________

b) the number of reduced-dosage nights ______________________

c) the number of usual-dosage nights ______________________

CHAPTER SIX

Establishing Sleep-Promoting Habits

William, a lifelong good sleeper, is the envy of all insomniacs. His bed is such a strong cue for sleep that he can drink cappucino at dinnertime, then get into an argument with his wife before bedtime, yet fall asleep as soon as his head hits the pillow. For Todd, an insomniac, the opposite is true. Due to years of insomnia, the bed has become so strongly associated with frustration and wakefulness that a kind of unconscious learning has set in. As a result, merely getting into bed triggers anxiety and wakefulness.

Just as we are creatures of habit, our sleep is a creation of habits. Like most insomniacs, Todd doesn't realize that many of the habits he has developed to cope with insomnia—such as going to bed early to catch up on sleep, resting in bed, and adopting the attitude "If I can't fall asleep, I'll just try harder"—actually exacerbate his insomnia. These habits weaken the brain's sleep system and become so strongly associated with wakefulness that they become powerful cues for insomnia.

In this chapter, you will learn sleep habits and behaviors that strengthen the brain's sleep system and create a positive association between the bed and sleep. Using these techniques to improve your sleep, mood, and energy, you will also enhance your confidence in your ability to change your sleep and your behavior.

Sleep-Scheduling Techniques

Sleep scheduling pertains to when you go to bed, when you get out of bed, and how much time you spend in bed. To use sleep-scheduling techniques to improve your sleep, you must first grasp two fundamental concepts: prior wakefulness and sleep efficiency.

Prior Wakefulness and Sleep Efficiency

Prior wakefulness refers to the number of hours that have elapsed from the time you rise in the morning until you turn off the lights at bedtime to go to sleep. Our sleep system follows a basic principle: the greater the amount of prior wakefulness, the greater the brain's pressure for sleep and the better we sleep.

The reason is well documented. With more prior wakefulness, we increase our exposure to sunlight and generate more physical activity, which, in turn, cause our body temperature to rise and fall more. As a result, our sleep system is strengthened and we sleep better. Therefore, the earlier you get out of bed and the later you go to bed, the more prior wakefulness you accrue and the better you will sleep. You will fall asleep faster, produce more sound sleep with fewer and shorter wake-ups, and sleep more hours.

Sleep efficiency is the ratio of time asleep divided by time spent in bed, or:

$$\frac{\text{Time Asleep}}{\text{Time in Bed}}$$

Recall from your 60-Second Sleep Diary that time in bed refers to the time elapsed from "lights out" at bedtime until you rise in the morning. So, if you spend eight hours in bed at night and sleep six hours, your sleep efficiency is 75 percent. On average, good sleepers exhibit a sleep efficiency of 90 percent—they are awake only 10 percent of the time they are in bed. In comparison, poor sleepers typically average 65 percent sleep efficiency—they are awake one-third of the time they are in bed.

You might think that the best measure for distinguishing normal sleep from insomnia is the amount of sleep. Actually, sleep efficiency is a better discriminator. Sleep efficiency also plays a primary role in learning to sleep poorly. Why? Because good sleepers are asleep most of the time they are in bed. As a result, the bed becomes a strong cue for sleep.

Insomniacs, however, are awake, usually tense and frustrated, for about one-third of the time that they are in bed. Consequently, the bed becomes a strong cue for wakefulness and frustration. In fact, because some insomniacs are awake in their bed more than they are asleep, the bed becomes a stronger cue for wakefulness than sleep! By learning to improve sleep efficiency, the bed will become a stronger cue for sleep, and your sleep will improve as a result.

One way to improve sleep efficiency is to learn to increase the time that you are asleep. Since all the techniques in this program are designed to help you fall asleep more easily, wake up less often and for shorter periods of time, and fall back to sleep more easily, they will improve sleep efficiency. The other way to improve sleep efficiency is to reduce time in bed. We will return to this idea later.

A Regular Rising Time

In an effort to make up for lost sleep, many insomniacs sleep in on weekends or after a bad night of sleep. Although this strategy may work in the short run by providing a few hours of extra sleep or bed rest, it actually contributes to insomnia in the long run for several reasons.

Recall that the body-temperature rhythm starts to rise in the morning when we get out of bed, become active, and allow sunlight to enter our eyes. If you sleep later on weekends or after a bad night of sleep, you delay the rise in your body-temperature rhythm because you delay physical activity and exposure to sunlight. If the elevation in your body temperature is delayed by a few hours, the drop in your temperature in the evening will also be delayed by the same amount of time. Therefore, if you try to go to bed at your normal time, you won't be able to fall asleep because your body temperature will be too elevated.

Sleeping later on weekends is the primary cause of Sunday-night insomnia, which is common among insomniacs and even affects good sleepers. Although you might think that Sunday-night insomnia is caused by the mental adjustment of the ending of the weekend and the beginning of the workweek, it is often due to later bedtimes and wake-up times on the weekend, which cause a delay in the body-temperature rhythm. When we try to go to sleep on Sunday night, we have more difficulty falling asleep because body temperature is still too high.

Although you can compensate for sleeping later on weekends by going to bed later on Sunday night (which gives your body temperature more time to fall), most insomniacs do just the opposite; they go to bed earlier in an attempt to get a good night's sleep for the beginning of the workweek.

The disruption in sleep caused by sleeping later on weekends or after a bad night of sleep is the same process involved in jet lag. Jet lag is caused by crossing time zones rapidly, which alters both the timing of our exposure to sunlight and our body-temperature rhythm. For example, imagine that you live in Boston and normally go to bed at 11:00 P.M. and rise at 7:00 A.M. If you fly to Denver and stay there for a few days, your body temperature will begin to rise and fall two hours later, because the sun rises and sets two hours later in Denver relative to Boston. Then, when you return to Boston and try to go to sleep at 11:00 P.M. Boston time, your body-temperature rhythm says its 9:00 P.M. Denver time and you will have more difficulty falling asleep.

By sleeping later on weekends or after a poor night of sleep, you delay your exposure to sunlight and induce jet lag without ever getting on an airplane! Just as some people's sleep is sensitive to a one-hour jet lag, some insomniacs are sensitive to even a one-hour variation in their rising time.

Sleeping in on weekends or after a bad night's sleep also causes difficulty staying asleep. By sleeping later on a given day and then attempting to go to bed at your normal time that night, you reduce your normal amount of prior wakefulness and minimize the rise and fall in your body-temperature rhythm. As a result, you will weaken your sleep system and have more difficulty staying asleep.

Therefore, sleep-scheduling rule number 1: *get out of bed around the same time every day, including weekends, no matter how little or poorly you have slept.* You should determine your preferred rising time, then set an alarm clock so that you stay within half an hour of that rising time every day. Planning enjoyable early morning activities such as reading the newspaper, exercising, walking the dog, or taking a walk will increase the likelihood that you will get out of bed at a consistent time. You should track the consistency of your rising time using the Weekly Progress Summary described at the end of this chapter.

If you have a poor night's sleep and feel you must sleep in to catch up, limit yourself to one extra hour and expose yourself to sunlight as soon as you get out of bed to help your body temperature rise. You can also compensate for sleeping in by delaying your bedtime that night; the delay will increase prior wakefulness and give your body temperature more time to fall.

By establishing a regular arising time, you will fall asleep more easily, sleep more deeply, and wake less often and for shorter periods of time. You will also improve your sleep efficiency, make the bed a stronger cue for sleep, and sleep even better as a result.

Reducing Time Allotted for Sleep

Another common coping strategy among insomniacs is to go to bed early in order to get a head start on sleep, to increase the likelihood of being asleep by a certain time, or to catch up on lost sleep or bed rest. Some insomniacs also go to bed early simply to escape boredom.

Instead of leading to increased sleep time, however, going to bed early actually exacerbates insomnia. This is because of a simple principle: the earlier you go to bed and the more time you spend in bed, the more you reduce prior wakefulness, weaken the sleep system, and exacerbate insomnia. In the long run, increased time in bed also contributes to reduced sleep efficiency and makes the bed a stronger cue for wakefulness.

Therefore, sleep-scheduling rule number 2: *reduce your time in bed so that it more closely matches the amount of sleep you are averaging per night.* For example, suppose your sleep diaries indicate that you are averaging five hours of sleep and you are spending eight hours in bed. Your goal would be to reduce your time in bed so that it more closely approximates five hours. This can be accomplished by going to bed later, getting up earlier, or a combination of both.

Your should determine your maximum allowable time in bed by simply adding one hour to your average sleep time. So if you are averaging six hours of sleep, your time in bed should be limited to a maximum of seven hours. (However, don't restrict time in bed to less than five and a half hours; otherwise, you won't be able to obtain core sleep.)

You should also determine your earliest allowable bedtime by starting from your desired wake-up time and subtracting your maximum allowable time in bed. For example, if you have determined that your maximum allowable time in bed should be six hours and you want to get out of bed by 6:00 A.M. each day, you should not get into bed before midnight no matter how tired you feel.

Contrary to what you may think, reducing time in bed will not reduce sleep time. Rather, it will increase prior wakefulness, strengthen the sleep system, and therefore increase your sleep time. Sleep efficiency will also improve and your bed will become a stronger cue for sleep.

Reducing time in bed is only temporary until your sleep efficiency improves to 85 percent (which is near the average normal-sleeper range of 90 percent). Once you have maintained a sleep efficiency of at least 85 percent for two weeks, you can increase time in bed by fifteen minutes each week so long as you maintain that level of sleep efficiency. Eventually, you will reach a point at which you are obtaining the amount of sleep that is satisfactory to you. Begin tracking your sleep efficiency using the Weekly Progress Summary described at the end of this chapter.

To help you reduce time in bed so that it more closely matches your average sleep time, here are other suggestions:

1. Since you will be going to bed later, getting up earlier, or both, view this extra time out of bed as an opportunity to accomplish other things or engage in pleasurable activities.

2. If you find it difficult to go to bed later because you feel too fatigued, use physical activity—such as taking a walk or completing a household chore or project—a few hours before your new, later bedtime to ward off fatigue. If you watch television or are a "couch potato" the entire evening, it will be harder to delay your bedtime.

3. Your sleep system does not operate like a switch that can simply be turned on. That's why many insomniacs can't work and think at full speed until 11:00 P.M. and then expect to fall asleep by 11:30 and sleep soundly.

It is necessary to wind down gradually in the hour before bedtime by engaging in relaxing activities such as light reading, a hobby, or listening to music. During this wind-down period, avoid stimulating activities such as telephone calls, arguments or emotional discussions, work-related activities, computers, bill-paying, or unpleasant television programs.

However, if you are so relaxed during the wind-down period that you can't stay out of bed until your new delayed bedtime, engage in occasional, light physical activity to ward off fatigue—walk around during television commercials or after every tenth page of a book.

4. If you decide to reduce time in bed by rising earlier in the morning, pair your earlier rising time with an activity such as exercising, walking the dog, or drinking a cup of coffee while reading the newspaper. These strategies will help you feel more alert and will increase the likelihood that you will stick with your earlier rising time.

Napping

Ever wondered why you feel a midafternoon slump in your mood and alertness, especially after a poor night of sleep? Many people believe this slump is caused by eating a heavy lunch. However, in reality, this occurs because we were meant to have a midafternoon nap.

Several lines of evidence, including the universal tendency of toddlers and the elderly to nap in the afternoon, and the afternoon nap of siesta cultures, have led sleep researchers to the same conclusion: nature intended that we take a nap in the middle of the day. This biological readiness to fall asleep in midafternoon, which coincides with a slight drop in body temperature and occurs regardless of whether or not we eat lunch, is almost as strong as the nighttime pressure to fall asleep. It is present even in good sleepers who are well rested. Sleep researchers have also discovered that the afternoon dip in mood and alertness is associated with poorer performance, particularly after a night of sleep loss.

A midday nap is an integral part of the daily routine of many cultures, particularly those near the equator. This suggests that napping may have been part of an evolutionary mechanism to get us out of the hot midday sun. However, because the urge for a nap is appreciably weaker than the need to sleep at night, it can be suppressed (or masked by caffeine). Also, because naps conflict with work schedules, they are becoming less common in industrialized societies (with the exception of college students and the elderly, who have more regular opportunities to nap). Unfortunately, this decline in napping may be causing poorer afternoon alertness and performance.

Research on napping suggests that an afternoon nap as short as ten minutes can enhance alertness, mood, and mental performance, especially after a night of poor sleep. In one study on napping, pilots on long-distance airplane flights who were allowed to take a brief nap in the cockpit (when they weren't flying the plane) were less fatigued, more alert and vigilant, and performed better. There is also some evidence to suggest that naps may have other health benefits. In a study conducted in Greece, naps were correlated with a 30 percent reduction in the incidence of coronary heart disease.

If you have an opportunity for an afternoon nap, particularly after a poor night of sleep, take one; you will feel more alert and energetic afterwards. However, make sure you limit your nap to forty-five minutes and don't take it later than 4:00 P.M.; otherwise, you may enter deep sleep, which may cause you to feel groggy for a period of time after the nap and reduce the pressure for sleep that night.

Interestingly, there is evidence that simply resting in the mid-afternoon can improve mood. Sleep itself may not be the crucial factor in the effects of afternoon naps on improving mood; what may be important is an afternoon period of relaxation common to both resting and napping. We'll return to this idea when we explore relaxation techniques.

Stimulus-Control Techniques

Many of our daily behaviors are influenced by learned cues, or stimuli, in our environment. For example, through years of associating movie theaters with popcorn, many people have had the experience of eating a large meal, then going to a movie and finding themselves desiring a box of popcorn. This is due to the fact that, through repeated associations, the movie theater has become a learned cue for eating popcorn. This is an example of a behavior that is under stimulus control.

Other examples of stimulus control include feeling hungry when the clock says noon or whenever we walk into the kitchen; feeling anxious when the telephone rings in the middle of the night but not when it rings during the day; or smokers reaching for a cigarette whenever they drink a cup of coffee. In each of these situations, environmental cues influence behavior.

Just as many of our daytime behaviors are under stimulus control, so, too, is our sleep. For good sleepers, years of good sleep have made the bed a strong cue for sleep. In fact, it is not uncommon for good sleepers to go to bed with the intention of watching television or reading for a while, yet quickly finding themselves struggling to stay awake.

For poor sleepers, the opposite is true. They have lain awake for so many nights that the bed and bedroom have become strong cues for sleeplessness. As a result, just getting into bed triggers a learned arousal response and wakefulness. In fact, it is not uncommon for insomniacs to find themselves falling asleep in front of the television in the living room, yet when they get into their bed to go to sleep, they become wide awake.

Insomniacs engage in many behaviors that make the bed a cue for wakefulness. Some use their bedroom to watch television, talk on the phone, review work-related material, study, or solve problems with their spouse. Others go to bed not because they feel drowsy but because their spouse is going to bed, which strengthens the association between the bed and wakefulness.

Another behavior that makes the bed a cue for wakefulness is trying to force sleep in the belief that "If I try a little harder, sleep will eventually come." However, we can't force sleep. In fact, attempting to force sleep backfires and creates more physical and mental arousal, which strengthens the wakefulness system.

The effect of trying to sleep was demonstrated in a study in which some subjects were asked to fall asleep as fast as possible, with a cash prize for the most successful attempt, while others were simply asked to fall asleep as usual. The subjects who were offered the cash prize took three times as long to fall asleep. As this study demonstrated, trying to fall asleep causes increased mental and physical arousal in the form of faster brain waves, heart rate, breathing rate, and greater muscle tension. This makes it harder to fall asleep and contributes to associating the bed with wakefulness.

Stimulus-control procedures, which were originally developed by Dr. Richard Bootzin, are designed to help you unlearn the connection between the bed and insomnia. To make these procedures easier to implement, I have modified Dr. Bootzin's original techniques slightly. This modified version will also make it easier for you to associate your bed with drowsiness and sleep. Here are the basic steps:

Step 1. Use the bedroom for sleep and sexual activity only. Do not use the bedroom to watch television, work, study, or talk on the telephone. If reading or watching television in bed helps you fall asleep, limit these activities to twenty to thirty minutes so that you don't end up reading or watching television for long periods of time in the hope that you will induce sleep. (If necessary, set a timer to turn off the light or television so that you aren't awakened as easily if you fall asleep.) Your goal is to associate your bedroom with drowsiness and sleep, not wakefulness.

Step 2. Since your goal is to associate the bed with sleep, make sure you feel drowsy when you turn the lights off to go to sleep. Otherwise, you will be more likely to lie awake, think, and try to force sleep. Since you will be getting up earlier or going to bed later to reduce time in bed, you will naturally feel drowsier at bedtime.

Also, learn to identify your internal cues for drowsiness (eyelids dropping, head nodding, yawning, reading the same line in a book several times and not understanding it) rather than relying on external cues such as the clock, your bed partner's bedtime, or the end of the evening news. Your goal is to associate your bed with drowsiness.

Step 3. If you don't fall asleep within twenty to thirty minutes, or if you awaken during the night and don't fall back to sleep within that time, don't lie in bed tossing and turning (since focusing on the clock only heightens anxiety about falling asleep, the time limit should be estimated). Instead, either go to another room or sit up in bed and engage in a quiet, relaxing activity such as watching television or reading a book, magazine, or catalog until you are drowsy, then attempt to go to sleep again. Repeat this process as often as necessary until you fall asleep.

Staying in bed and reading or watching television when you can't sleep is all right as long as you go back to sleep in less than one hour; otherwise, you will associate the bed with wakefulness. If you go to another room when you can't sleep, don't allow yourself to fall asleep on the couch or you will end up teaching yourself that the couch is the only place where you can fall asleep.

You may be tempted to simply lie in bed when you can't sleep in the hope that "if I give it just a few more minutes, I'm bound to fall asleep" or "if I read when I can't sleep, I will just become more wide awake." However, you need to realize that the longer you lie in bed tossing and turning and trying to sleep, the longer you will lie awake.

You may also be concerned that reading in bed or getting out of bed when you can't sleep will disrupt your partner. Most partners will endure this minor inconvenience if your sleep and mood improve as a result. Tossing and turning is more disruptive to most partners than reading in bed or getting out of bed.

Finally, make certain that you have relaxing activities to engage in when you can't sleep; otherwise, you will become bored and frustrated, which will exacerbate insomnia.

With repeated practice, stimulus-control procedures will teach you to fall asleep more easily and to associate your bed with drowsiness and sleep instead of trying to sleep. Consequently, your bed will become a stronger cue for sleep instead of wakefulness, as in the case of one patient.

Michael came to my program averaging about two hours of waking time during the middle of the night. He routinely used his bed to review work-related materials or watch television and usually tossed and turned when he couldn't fall back to sleep during the night.

Michael began to practice stimulus-control techniques each night: he stopped using his bedroom as an office and as the primary room for watching television, and he learned to read a book when he didn't fall back to sleep within twenty minutes.

It wasn't easy, but Michael stuck with the stimulus-control procedures. Although his sleep did not improve much during the first week, he noticed improvement by the second week. After four weeks of consistently practicing the procedures, Michael was falling back to sleep within twenty minutes on most nights and felt a lot more relaxed about his sleep.

Your Week Two Progress Summary

Sleep-scheduling and stimulus-control techniques require effort and persistence and may require at least one week before you notice an improvement. The result of significantly improved sleep is well worth the effort. With continued practice, these techniques will become easier and more "automatic" to implement.

To help track your use of these techniques and their beneficial effects on your sleep, your Week Two Progress Summary is included at the end of this chapter. Take a moment to review it. Like the Week One Progress Summary, it should be completed after you review your seven sleep diaries for this week.

As you will see, the Week Two Progress Summary is similar to that for week one, for it contains items for assessing your current sleep pattern, sleep-medication use, and your use of cognitive restructuring techniques. It also contains new items to help you assess your average sleep time, time in bed, sleep efficiency, wake-up time, sleep quality, and your consistency in using sleep-scheduling and stimulus-control techniques.

After completing the Week Two Progress Summary, compare it to your Week One Progress Summary. You will probably note more nights of good sleep, core sleep, and reduced medication and fewer insomnia nights. Because the consistency with which you practice sleep-scheduling and stimulus-control techniques is directly related to improvement in your sleep, inspect your compliance with these techniques, which you will record in the progress summary. If sleep is not improving consistently, you are probably not practicing these techniques consistently and need to make a greater effort to do so.

You Can Change Your Behavior

By successfully using the techniques described in this chapter, you will accomplish much more than just improving your sleep. You will empower yourself with the knowledge that the key to conquering insomnia resides within you. You will also demonstrate to yourself the ability to change your behavior. This knowledge will increase confidence, optimism, and self-esteem, and provide a greater sense of control over your life.

WEEK TWO PROGRESS SUMMARY

1. Assess your sleep pattern this week by noting:
   a) the number of good nights of sleep ____________________
   b) the number of nights of core sleep (five and a half hours or more) ____________________
   c) the number of insomnia nights ____________________

2. On how many daily sleep diaries did you record a positive sleep thought? ____________________

3. How often did you mentally practice cognitive restructuring this week (circle one)?
   regularly
   occasionally
   never

4. Assess your sleep-medication use this week by noting:
   a) the number of medication-free nights ____________________
   b) the number of reduced-dosage nights ____________________
   c) the number of usual-dosage nights ____________________

5. Track your sleep efficiency by calculating:
   a) your average sleep time (number of hours per night) ____________________
   b) your average time in bed (number of hours per night) ____________________
   c) your average sleep efficiency (your average sleep time divided by your average time in bed) ____________________

6. Track your sleep quality and the consistency of your rising time by noting:

a) your average sleep-quality rating from your sleep diaries ______________________

b) the number of days you arose within half an hour of your desired rising time ______________________

7. How often did you practice sleep-scheduling and stimulus-control techniques this week (circle one)?

regularly

occasionally

never

CHAPTER SEVEN

Lifestyle and Environmental Factors That Affect Sleep

Many of our lifestyle practices affect our sleep. In this chapter, we will explore how to use exercise, sunlight, and a host of other factors to improve sleep. We will also examine how to create the optimal sleep environment.

Many of these practices will not just improve sleep; they can also change your life in significant and fundamental ways. By implementing them, you will live a longer, healthier, happier life, and they will contribute to a healthier self-image and better quality of life.

Exercise for Better Sleep and Health

The Consequences of a Sedentary Lifestyle

Our evolution over tens of thousands of years involved regular physical activity. Indeed, our early ancestors' day-to-day survival required physical activity in the form of hunting and gathering food. Daily physical activity was required later in our evolution to plant, sow, and harvest crops.

Yet consider now, in a remarkably short period of time, we have dramatically reduced our level of physical activity. Although there are many reasons, indoor work environments, computers, labor-saving devices, automobiles, and televisions are the primary culprits. These modern technological advances were intended to make life easier; in reality they have led to a mechanized lifestyle in which we sit at desks, in cars, or in front of the television set. We didn't evolve to inhabit the couch, yet many of us don't even change the channels on our televisions or open our garage doors ourselves.

Despite the public awareness of the negative consequences of a sedentary lifestyle, physical inactivity is epidemic in the United States. At least 25 percent of adults (and an alarming number of children) are inactive and overweight. Consequently, a significant percentage of Americans have chronic medical problems directly related to physical inactivity and obesity, including heart disease, high blood pressure, diabetes, and some types of cancer.

It is not surprising that individuals with these health problems are also at significantly increased risk of dying prematurely. At least one in ten deaths in the United States each year is attributable to a lack of physical activity.

The Many Benefits of Exercise

If sedentary adults would adopt a more physically active lifestyle, they would experience a wide array of physical and mental benefits, including:

- Weight loss, improved physical appearance, and positive body image
- Lessened anxiety, stress, and depression
- Improved mood, energy, and sense of well-being
- Improved self-esteem, confidence, and feelings of self-control
- Improved health, longevity, and quality of life
- Reduced pain and disability

Regular exercise enhances health by improving cardiovascular functioning, bone density, and immune functioning, and by reducing blood pressure and cholesterol. People who are physically active are much less likely to suffer from coronary heart disease, hypertension, diabetes, osteoporosis, obesity, back problems, and colon cancer.

Exercise also improves psychological functioning. Exercise is an outlet for the body's excessive tension, providing a healthy way to release anger and anxiety. Exercise has a tranquilizing effect that reduces anxiety more effectively than many antianxiety medications. Studies have found that the tranquilizing effect follows within five to ten minutes of completing exercise and lasts for at least four hours. Therefore, physically active people are less likely to develop mental health problems such as anxiety and depression.

Exercise is an effective treatment for people suffering from depression. In one study, mild to moderately depressed people reported feeling better within one week of beginning an exercise program; they also improved more over time than mild to moderately depressed people who received either short- or long-term psychotherapy. Exercise also improves emotional well-being by enhancing self-esteem. People who exercise feel better about themselves and their bodies. And, because exercise improves appearance, others' compliments about physical improvements from exercise further enhance one's self-esteem.

Exercise has such a wide range of physical and mental benefits that, if it were a pill, it would undoubtedly be the most widely prescribed of all medications. It is amazing that, despite this evidence and the public's apparent acceptance of the importance of physical activity, millions of American adults remain sedentary.

Exercise as a Sleep Aid

Two findings about exercise are particularly relevant to insomniacs. One, insomniacs lead more sedentary lives than good sleepers. The lack of physical activity can contribute to insomnia by inhibiting the daily rise and fall of the body-temperature rhythm. As a result, many people get caught in a cycle of insomnia, reduced energy and physical activity, and worsened insomnia.

Two, exercise improves sleep by producing a significant rise in body temperature, followed by a compensatory drop a few hours later. The drop in body temperature, which persists for two to four hours after exercise, makes it easier to fall asleep and stay asleep.

The beneficial effect of exercise on sleep is greatest when exercise occurs within three to six hours of bedtime. Exercising less than three hours before bedtime, however, can make it more difficult to fall asleep, for body temperature may then be too elevated.

Exercise also improves sleep because it is a physical stressor to the body. The brain compensates for physical stress by increasing deep sleep. Therefore, we sleep more deeply and soundly after exercise. Exercise may also improve sleep because people often exercise outdoors during the day, which increases exposure to sunlight. We will shortly explore how exposure to sunlight improves sleep by synchronizing our body-temperature rhythm.

Mary Ellen was one of my patients whose story illustrates the beneficial effect of exercise on sleep. She is a forty-year-old housewife who came to my insomnia program complaining of difficulty falling and staying asleep. Mary Ellen's sleep diaries revealed that she required an average of one hour per night to fall asleep and that her nighttime awakenings averaged ninety minutes.

Because she was sedentary, Mary Ellen was advised to begin an exercise program. She chose to walk briskly for thirty minutes late in the day. Within a few weeks she was falling asleep within thirty minutes each night, and she reduced the frequency and length of her nighttime awakenings by about 50 percent. She felt more rested; her mood and daily functioning began to improve.

Although exercise alone didn't cure Mary Ellen's insomnia, it had a significant positive effect on her sleep.

In another example of the beneficial effect of exercise on sleep, Stanford University School of Medicine researchers studied the effects of exercise on the sleep patterns of adults aged fifty-five to seventy-five who were sedentary and troubled by insomnia. These adults were asked to exercise for twenty to thirty minutes every other day in the afternoon by walking, engaging in low-impact aerobics, and riding a stationary bicycle. The result? The time required to fall asleep was reduced by half, and sleep time increased by almost one hour.

Physical Activity Versus Intense Exercise

With all the benefits associated with exercise, why do so few American adults exercise? There are many reasons; some of the more common ones include:

> **"I am too busy and don't have the time."**
> **"I don't like discomfort or sweat."**
> **"Exercise is too boring or is too much work."**
> **"The weather's bad."**
> **"I don't enjoy exercise."**

Perhaps the major reason people don't exercise is the misperception that exercise means sweat-soaked, exhausting, torturous physical exertion. This concept is partially the result of an overemphasis on the importance of engaging in twenty to thirty minutes of high-intensity exercise three to five times per week, which has discouraged many.

New scientific evidence clearly indicates that moderate physical activity, not just intense exercise, provides substantial health benefits. New guidelines involving a gentler, easier exercise program of daily physical activity were recommended in 1996 by the surgeon general and by experts. The new program encourages adults to become and remain active. The guidelines recommend at least thirty minutes of moderate-intensity physical activity on most, if not all, days. This activity can come in the form of many of our normal daily activities: washing the car, taking the stairs instead of the elevator, or riding a bicycle instead of driving.

These activities can be broken up into several shorter sessions that, during the day, add up to thirty minutes—enough physical activity to expend about 200 calories daily. The total amount of activity is more important than whether it involves intense physical exercise or moderate-intensity activity.

The good news: you don't have to join a health club, use a Stairmaster, do aerobics, or work up a sweat to obtain health benefits from exercise!

Listed below are moderate-intensity physical activities:

- Home care, general cleaning, mowing the lawn with a nonriding mower
- Home repair and painting, gardening, raking leaves
- Climbing steps
- Playing actively with children
- Washing the car, windows, or floors
- Pushing a stroller
- Walking briskly, three to four miles per hour
- Bicyling for pleasure or transportation
- Table tennis or doubles tennis
- Golf (carrying or pulling clubs), fishing, canoeing

Here are some examples of activities that are more vigorous and will produce even greater health benefits:

- Walking briskly uphill or with a load
- Hand mowing a lawn or moving furniture
- Day hiking or backpacking
- Dancing or fast bicycling
- Vigorous swimming
- Basketball, singles tennis, running
- Racquetball, ski machine, treadmill, Stairmaster
- Aerobics or cross-country skiing

Experts agree that most adults do not need to see their physician before beginning a moderate-intensity physical activity program. However, it is a good idea to build up levels of physical activity by starting with low-intensity activities for short durations a few times a week, then gradually increasing the duration and frequency.

Those who plan to start more vigorous physical exercise or who have a chronic health problem should first consult their physician to plan a safe, effective program. Vigorous exercise should also be preceded and followed by a few minutes of stretching to work out muscle tightness and reduce the risk of muscle injury.

How to Succeed at Exercise

In addition to focusing on moderate physical activity, these guidelines will increase the likelihood of becoming and remaining physically active:

- Choose activities that you enjoy and that give a sense of satisfaction. What works for some is torture for others. Some people listen to music or watch television while they exercise to make it more enjoyable.
- View physical activity and exercise as a break from your daily routine. Use the time as an opportunity to focus on your surroundings and the present rather than the past, the future, and problems and worries.
- Focus on the activity, not your performance (for example, how fast or how many miles you have walked).
- Vary the types of activities and exercise that you engage in. Having several options relieves boredom.
- Avoid labor-saving devices such as riding lawn mowers, leaf blowers, remote controls, and chain saws.
- Exercise with your family or friends and you will be more likely to receive support and encouragement and view exercise as "quality" time. Bicycling is a great example of family exercise.
- Expect occasional periods when you can't exercise, such as during an illness or when you are injured or not feeling well.
- During periods of extreme heat or cold, move indoors or change the timing of exercise to adjust to your environment. During the winter months, many adults have turned to mall walking as a regular form of exercise. Many

malls now open very early to allow walkers to beat the shoppers and begin their day with a brisk walk. Because malls are air-conditioned, they are also ideal places to exercise on hot summer days.

Can't Exercise? Try a Bath

Several studies have demonstrated that, like exercise, a hot bath causes a rise and fall in body temperature that can make it easier to fall asleep and stay asleep. The bath must be hot and kept hot for about twenty-five minutes. Also, because the temperature drop after a bath occurs more quickly than after exercise, the bath should be taken about two hours before bedtime (baths taken too close to bedtime can make it harder to fall asleep because body temperature may be too elevated).

A hot bath can aid sleep but it is usually not as effective as exercise at improving sleep, for baths do not cause as much of a rise and fall in body temperature. However, a hot bath is a great way to relax before bedtime and a good substitute on days when you can't exercise.

Exercising the Brain

Just as we need to be physically active to sleep well, we also need to be mentally active (though not at bedtime). Boredom can reduce the pressure for sleep and contribute to insomnia, for the brain is not being stimulated. Some people also attempt to escape boredom by spending more time in bed, which, as we have explored, contributes to insomnia.

To alleviate boredom, don't sit at home, a couch potato, watching television. Instead, take courses, learn to use a computer, investigate new hobbies or activities, read books, travel, socialize. Studies have shown that mental and intellectual stimulation increase the pressure for sleep. You will also add some excitement to your life!

Improve Sleep and Mood with Bright Light

The Sunlight-Sleep Connection

As we have seen, sleep and body temperature are directly influenced by the effect of the daily cycles of light and darkness on melatonin, a naturally occurring hormone found in the brain. When sunlight enters the eyes, melatonin levels decrease, which signals body temperature to rise and promotes wakefulness. Darkness causes melatonin levels to increase and body temperature to fall, which promotes sleep.

Consider how, for almost our entire evolution as hunter-gatherers, we were exposed to the natural cycle of sunlight during the day and darkness at night. However, with the advent of modern technology, we have significantly altered our exposure to light and darkness. Studies have shown that, no matter where people live, they obtain only one hour of sunlight on average during the day. The nighttime lighting of urban environments means that many people also don't receive exposure to true darkness anymore.

The main reason we obtain so little sunlight is that most of us work indoors. A brightly lit room has about 500 luxes of light (a lux is the equivalent of the light from one candle) compared to 10,000 luxes at sunrise and 100,000 at noon on a summer day. To the brain, spending the day indoors is equivalent to spending the day in darkness!

By reducing our exposure to bright natural light and true darkness, melatonin secretion and the body-temperature rhythm are altered, which can exacerbate sleep difficulties. That's why up to 90 percent of blind people experience sleep problems. Likewise, lack of exposure to bright light can also adversely affect daytime mood, energy, and alertness level. For example, studies show that mood and energy are poorest during the winter months, which have the shortest days and therefore the least amount of sunlight. Furthermore, people in northern latitudes, where there is less sunlight in the wintertime, are more prone to seasonal affective disorder, which is characterized by depression and sleep disturbance in the winter months. Indeed, some scientists believe that the lack of exposure to sunlight may be contributing to an overall increase in mood disorders in the general population. Since lack of exposure to sunlight can disturb mood, it can also make it harder to cope with the daytime effects of insomnia.

Consequently, increased exposure to sunlight at certain times of the day can minimize sleep-onset insomnia and early morning awakenings. We have seen that sleep-onset insomnia is characterized by a body-temperature rhythm that falls too late at night. Because sunlight causes body temperature to rise, sleep-onset insomniacs can cause their body temperature to rise earlier and fall earlier, and therefore fall asleep more easily, by increasing exposure to early morning sunlight. This can be accomplished by using these basic strategies:

- Open the drapes or shades immediately upon awakening
- Eat breakfast near a sun-exposed window
- Avoid dark sunglasses in the morning
- Take an early morning walk

In contrast to sleep-onset insomnia, individuals who experience early morning awakenings often exhibit a body-temperature rhythm that rises too early in the morning. Several studies have shown that increasing exposure to evening bright light can minimize early morning awakenings by delaying the body-temperature rhythm so that it doesn't rise as soon. Simple techniques for increasing exposure to late-day sunlight include:

- Avoid dark sunglasses late in the day
- Take a late afternoon walk
- Sit near a sun-exposed window the hour before sunset
- Leave the drapes open until dark

Since bright light also improves energy and alertness, you may be able to tolerate the daytime effects of insomnia better by getting outside on your coffee break or lunch hour and thereby increasing your exposure to sunlight.

Artificial Bright Light: Bringing the Sun Indoors

Another method for increasing exposure to bright light is the use of artificial bright-light boxes. These devices contain special bulbs that emit 5,000–10,000 luxes of light, which is equivalent to a sunrise or sunset. They are used for about thirty minutes while reading or watching television to increase early or late exposure to bright light. Several studies have demonstrated that using bright-light boxes in the evening can delay the body-temperature rhythm and effectively minimize early morning insomnia.

By shifting body-temperature rhythms, bright-light boxes also seem to minimize the sleep disturbances associated with jet lag and shift work. One company has even developed a baseball-type cap that contains bright lights. When traveling, the caps can be programmed to turn on and off at certain times to adjust to another time zone, thereby minimizing jet lag. Bright-light boxes are also used as a primary treatment for seasonal affective disorder, and some companies are using them to increase the alertness of night shift workers during the early morning hours.

Light boxes can be rented from medical supply companies or purchased from an increasing number of manufacturers. Some insurance companies even reimburse the cost of light boxes if they are prescribed by a physician.

How Caffeine, Nicotine and Alcohol Can Disturb Sleep

Caffeine: Society's Stimulant

Caffeine is the most widely used drug in the world. Found primarily in coffee, tea, and cola, caffeine is a stimulant that speeds up brain waves, increases heart rate and blood pressure, and promotes alertness and reduces fatigue. These stimulant effects, which work in as little as fifteen minutes and can last for six or more hours, can also disturb sleep. Consequently, insomniacs who use caffeine to counteract afternoon or early evening fatigue can get caught in a cycle of caffeine use and insomnia.

Caffeine can also produce daytime anxiety symptoms such as nervousness, irritability, shakiness, and sweaty palms, and can also cause more frequent nighttime urination, which interrupts sleep. Because, as we will note shortly, nicotine is also a stimulant, individuals who smoke and drink coffee make it twice as difficult to fall asleep or stay asleep.

We vary greatly in our sensitivity to the stimulant effects of caffeine. Some of us have a natural tolerance to it and can fall asleep after drinking two cups in the evening, while others have trouble sleeping after drinking one cup in the afternoon. Insomniacs are more likely to experience sleep disturbance from caffeine due to an overly sensitive sleep system, as are elderly adults, who metabolize caffeine more slowly.

If caffeine is consumed in large-enough quantities, it can also lead to dependency and withdrawal symptoms such as headaches, anxiety, irritability, and insomnia. A seven-ounce cup of coffee contains an average of 110 mg of caffeine (in comparison, a cup of tea and a twelve-ounce soft drink contain about 50 mg each), but the average cup of coffee sold today by coffee specialty stores is twelve ounces, which means that if you drink three of these cups of coffee a day you may be consuming more than 500 mg of caffeine. This can lead to dependency and withdrawal symptoms that can disturb sleep.

Does all this mean that insomniacs should give up caffeine altogether? Probably not, for drinking one or two cups of coffee in the morning is unlikely to affect nighttime sleep. However, since caffeine's stimulant effects may affect some individuals for six hours or longer, and the withdrawal effects for people who are dependent upon caffeine can last even longer, it should be avoided after lunchtime.

If you believe you are caffeine dependent, attempt to reduce caffeine intake gradually by mixing caffeinated coffee with decaffeinated (decaffeinated coffee actually contains about 2 mg of caffeine, which is not enough to affect sleep). This gradual approach to reducing caffeine consumption will minimize the likelihood of withdrawal symptoms such as headaches, jitteriness, and insomnia. Reducing caffeine consumption can also reduce daytime anxiety and nighttime awakenings due to frequent urination.

In addition to coffee, tea, and soft drinks, caffeine is also found in the following:

- Foods such as ice cream and yogurt, cocoa and chocolate
- Some analgesics, such as Anacin and Excedrin
- Some prescription migraine medications
- Many diet and cold remedies

One final word of caution about caffeine: make sure your children don't drink caffeinated beverages in the afternoon. When a child drinks a can of cola, the caffeine intake is comparable to four cups of coffee for an adult. As a result, your child may not be able to fall asleep at night.

Nicotine and Sleep

The issue of substance abuse is usually associated with illicit drugs such as heroin and cocaine. In reality, nicotine is more addictive and costly to society than such illegal drugs. Nicotine represents the nation's number one chemical-dependency problem.

Cigarette smoking is also more deadly than illicit drugs. Smoking is the leading cause of preventable disease and death in the United States, contributing to over 400,000 deaths annually, and it is directly linked to premature death from heart disease, emphysema, hypertension, stroke, diabetes, and many types of cancer.

Nicotine also harms sleep. The effects of nicotine are similar to those of caffeine and include faster brain waves, heart rate, and breathing rate, and increased amounts of stress hormones. These stimulant effects, which last for several hours after smoking a cigarette, can make it harder to fall asleep and stay asleep.

Smokers also experience nicotine-withdrawal effects during sleep that cause lighter sleep and more awakenings. Smoking also irritates the upper air passage and can exacerbate snoring and diminish sleep quality. That's why smokers sleep more poorly than nonsmokers and why insomnia ranks as one of the major health complaints of smokers. In short, smokers cannot expect to sleep well.

If you smoke, you will have the greatest beneficial effect on your sleep if you stop altogether. Numerous studies have shown that when smokers quit they sleep better in spite of temporary withdrawal symptoms such as restlessness, irritability, anxiety, difficulty concentrating, and headaches, which can persist for about ten days. Once the withdrawal symptoms end, sleep improves even more dramatically.

Only a small percentage of smokers quit permanently, and those who do usually do it "cold turkey." However, an increasing percentage are quitting successfully by using nicotine patches, which are substituted for cigarettes. The patches, which are placed on the skin and worn for most of the day, prevent the physical nicotine-withdrawal symptoms from occurring by administering nicotine through the skin in a gradual, decreasing dose.

Nicotine patches are effective in helping some smokers to quit. However, they are more effective when combined with behavioral strategies such as these:

- Gradually reducing the number of cigarettes smoked
- Selecting a target quit date
- Recognizing triggers for smoking (such as stress, eating, driving, caffeine, and alcohol) and substituting healthy behavioral alternatives such as the relaxation techniques described in part III
- Avoiding people or situations that encourage smoking
- Mentally reinforcing the consequences of smoking and the benefits of quitting
- Enlisting social support and reinforcement from family and friends

If you are a smoker, talk to your physician about these approaches. The National Cancer Institute, the American Heart Association, and the American Lung Association provide written materials that describe behavioral strategies for smoking cessation. If you can't quit, then try to eliminate smoking near bedtime or during the night. You will minimize the stimulant and withdrawal effects of nicotine and will sleep better.

Alcohol: The Nightcap That Causes Insomnia

Physicians used to prescribe a nightcap for insomnia, and many people still think that alcohol is a cure for sleeplessness. Although alcohol does relax some people enough that they fall asleep more easily, others find that it stimulates them and makes it more difficult to fall asleep.

Even if alcohol makes it easier to fall asleep, it can make sleep lighter and more fragmented, for it suppresses deep sleep. Alcohol also suppresses dream sleep, which results in dream sleep "rebound" in the form of intense dreaming or nightmares that can cause awakenings during the second half of the night.

Alcohol also disturbs sleep because, as it is metabolized during sleep, it produces mild withdrawal symptoms that cause sleep to become interrupted, shortened, and fragmented. These disruptions result in lighter sleep and more awakenings, particularly in the early morning. Alcohol also exacerbates snoring and sleep apnea because it relaxes the muscles in the throat. And remember: if you combine alcohol with sleeping pills, you are risking your life.

It requires about one and a half hours to metabolize one ounce of alcohol; the mild withdrawal effects last for another two to four hours. This means that a glass of wine with dinner will probably not affect sleep. However, one ounce of alcohol within two hours of bedtime or more than one ounce after dinner probably will disrupt sleep. Therefore, if you drink alcoholic beverages in the evening, you will minimize sleep problems if you limit yourself to one drink at least two hours before bedtime. If you are accustomed to having more than one drink in the evening, your sleep will improve if you cut back gradually to one.

Using alcohol to fall asleep also increases the risk of slipping into nightly alcohol use and becoming dependent upon it. In fact, 10 percent of all cases of alcoholism have been attributed to insomniacs who began using alcohol to aid sleep and then slipped into regular use.

Alcoholism can seriously disturb sleep. Alcoholics exhibit significant sleep disruptions that resemble those of older adults; these include diminished deep sleep, increased light sleep, and frequent awakenings. These sleep problems can last for months or years after alcoholics stop drinking, suggesting that chronic alcohol abuse may cause permanent and irreversible damage to the brain's sleep system.

If you think you are dependent on alcohol, you should talk with your physician about obtaining professional help.

The Food-Sleep Connection

Although there has been little research on the effects of food on sleep, it appears that certain types of food promote sleep while others inhibit it.

For example, foods such as bread, bagels, and crackers that are high in complex carbohydrates have a mild sleep-enhancing effect because they increase serotonin, a brain neurotransmitter that promotes sleep. In contrast, foods such as meat that are high in protein can inhibit sleep by blocking the synthesis of serotonin, making us feel more alert. These effects were demonstrated in a study in which people reported feeling more alert following a high-protein lunch and sleepier following a high-carbohydrate lunch.

If you want to fall asleep more easily, eat a high-carbohydrate snack and avoid high-protein foods in the hour or two before bedtime. If you desire to minimize nighttime awakenings, eat a carbohydrate snack immediately before bedtime, which will increase serotonin levels during the night and help you stay asleep. Having a light carbohydrate snack before bedtime will also ensure that your sleep isn't disturbed due to hunger.

Other types of foods can also disturb sleep and should be avoided before bedtime:

- Foods high in sugar and refined carbohydrates, which raise blood-sugar levels and can cause a burst of energy that disturbs sleep
- Foods that are likely to cause gas, heartburn, or indigestion, such as fatty or spicy foods, garlic-flavored foods, beans, cucumbers, and peanuts
- Monosodium glutamate (MSG), often found in Chinese food, which causes a stimulant reaction in some people

Because the digestive system slows at night, it is harder to digest late meals. The likelihood of indigestion increases, so avoid heavy meals before bedtime. Also reduce fluid intake after 8 P.M. and thus minimize the probability of waking up at night due to a full bladder.

Some research suggests that deficiencies in certain vitamins and minerals can also disrupt sleep. The research found that deficiencies in B vitamins and folic acid impair sleep; another study found that increasing dietary levels of B vitamins improves sleep. Deficiencies in calcium and magnesium, two minerals that produce calming effects on the brain and that are essential for normal sleep, can also disturb sleep. If you think that your diet is deficient in these substances, you may want to talk with your physician about modifying your diet or adding dietary supplements.

What about the use of herbal remedies as sleep aids? The most common herb used for insomnia is valerian root. Although some insomniacs find that this is effective as a sleep aid, others find that it has little or no effect. As is the case with most herbal remedies, no sound scientific studies have been conducted on valerian root. Scant information exists concerning its long-term side effects on health.

And what about the old adage that a glass of warm milk before bedtime improves sleep? Although this has never been substantiated scientifically, milk contains calcium and may therefore have a mild sleep-promoting effect. It's also likely that drinking warm milk creates a placebo effect that aids sleep.

How to Create the Optimal Sleep Environment

Just as our work and home environments affect our moods, our bedroom environment can affect our sleep. An uncomfortable bed or a room that is either too noisy, too hot, or too cold can disturb even the soundest sleeper. By keeping the following guidelines in mind, you can create the ideal sleep environment.

A Warm Room Can Keep You Awake

Room temperature can have a significant effect on sleep. Recall that insomnia is associated with a failure of body temperature to fall either at bedtime or during the night. Sleeping in a warm room will make it even harder for your body temperature to decrease. This will make it more difficult to fall asleep, and because deep sleep will also be reduced, nighttime awakenings will be more likely to occur. This explains why sleep is poorer in the summer months for the general population.

On the other hand, body temperature shows a more rapid drop in cooler rooms. In fact, the lower the room temperature at which we go to sleep, the greater the drop in body temperature and the easier it will be to fall asleep and stay asleep. That's why, when the weather cools down, it's common to hear weather forecasters say, "It's going to be great sleeping weather tonight."

Keep your room cool by turning the heat down, leaving a window open, or using a fan or air conditioner. If you have a partner who prefers a warmer bedroom, provide an extra blanket for that side of the bed.

Keep the Bedroom Dark and Quiet

Many types of noise such as traffic, loud music, a dripping faucet, a bed partner's snoring, a neighbor's barking dog, trains and airplanes, and neighbors can disturb sleep. Because insomniacs' sleep systems are more sensitive overall, sleep is more easily disrupted by noise. Older individuals, who are more sensitive to noise in general and whose sleep is lighter as a consequence of aging, are also more likely to experience noise-induced sleep disturbance.

There are a number of ways to minimize bedroom noise. Earplugs work well for many people. For others, the hum of a fan, an air conditioner, or a commercially available sound conditioner is useful. These devices work by blocking distracting noises and by producing constant, soothing sounds like water or rain that relax the brain and induce sleep. Using a fan or air conditioner in the summertime also allows you to sleep with the windows closed, which will reduce noise.

Listening to music at bedtime helps some people fall asleep. If you do so, make sure that you set a timer so that the music turns off after about forty-five minutes. Otherwise, you are more likely to wake up during the night, because music, like all sound, prevents us from entering deep sleep.

Our sleep is more susceptible to being disturbed by noise when we sleep in an unfamiliar place such as a friend or relative's home or a hotel room, particularly on the first night. Although sleep will usually improve on successive nights in a new place, be realistic and don't expect to sleep as well in these circumstances. Using the fan or the air conditioner in a hotel room is a simple and effective way to mask unwanted noise and improve sleep.

A bedroom that is insufficiently dark can also disturb sleep. Keep your bedroom dark by using drapes, heavy shades, or an eyeshade if necessary.

Your Bed Can Make a Difference

We go through up to a dozen posture shifts per night in which we awaken briefly, move, then quickly fall back to sleep. When we sleep with a partner, we also awaken briefly in response to their posture shifts. Even though many people think they sleep better with a partner, sleep is actually lighter, more restless, and more disturbed.

If you sleep with a partner, particularly one who is a restless sleeper, your sleep will be less disturbed if you switch to a bigger bed or twin beds. Think of it this way: you may not feel as intimate, but you will be less disturbed by your partner's movements, sleep more soundly, and wake less often. If your partner is a heavy snorer, separate bedrooms may be necessary if he or she is unwilling to seek medical treatment.

Bedding should also be comfortable and provide support. Beds that sag can disturb sleep by causing neck and back discomfort, while mattresses that are too hard can cause discomfort for people with arthritis. A simple way to create a firmer mattress is to place a sheet of half-inch plywood under it. Turning your mattress over and rotating it every six months can also be helpful. There is no evidence showing that sleep is different on a water bed rather than a regular mattress, so choose whichever is most comfortable for you.

Your Week Three Progress Summary

Like many of the techniques in this program, the lifestyle practices described in this chapter require some effort, persistence, and time to work. The techniques become easier with practice; by using them regularly you will be promoting a longer, healthier life.

To help track your use of these practices and their beneficial effects on your sleep, a Week Three Progress Summary is included at the end of this chapter. Like the Week One and Week Two summaries, it should be completed after you review your seven sleep diaries for the week.

The Week Three Progress Summary is similar to the Week Two summary; it contains the same items for assessing your current sleep pattern, sleep-medication use, and use of cognitive-restructuring, sleep-scheduling, and stimulus-control techniques. However, you will note that the Week Three Progress Summary also contains a new item for assessing your use of lifestyle practices as explored in this chapter.

If the progress summary indicates that you are not implementing these practices consistently, make a greater effort to do so—your sleep and health are worth it.

Now that you have finished the third week of this six-week program, it is appropriate to step back and assess the improvements you have made in your sleep. Notice that your progress summary contains a section that lists ten possible areas of improvement. After you have completed the Week Three Progress Summary, compare it to the Week One and Week Two summaries. Next, determine which of the ten areas of improvement apply to you, then check them off. This will help you to systematically track your improvement through the remainder of the program.

Remember, the degree of improvement in your sleep is directly related to how consistently you use these techniques, and by doing so, it is likely that you will experience positive changes in other areas of your life:

- Improved daytime mood, energy, and productivity
- Greater sense of control over sleep
- Increased sense of optimism, confidence, and self-esteem
- Greater sense of calm, more relaxation
- Improved sense of well-being
- Greater control over mind and body

Therefore, the progress summary also contains a section for summarizing these or any other positive changes you have experienced since beginning the program. By completing the summary each week, you will learn to recognize and reinforce positive changes. You will also become more empowered in the knowledge that you can change yourself and your life in more fundamental and powerful ways.

WEEK THREE PROGRESS SUMMARY

1. Assess your sleep pattern this week by noting:
a) the number of good nights of sleep ____________________
b) the number of nights or core sleep (five and a half hours or more) ____________________
c) the number of insomnia nights ____________________

2. On how many daily sleep diaries did you record a positive sleep thought? ____________________

3. How often did you mentally practice cognitive restructuring this week (circle one)?
regularly
occasionally
never

4. Assess your sleep-medication use this week by noting:
a) the number of medication-free nights ____________________
b) the number of reduced-dosage nights ____________________
c) the number of usual-dosage nights ____________________

5. Track your sleep efficiency by calculating:
a) your average sleep time (number of hours per night) ____________________
b) your average time in bed (number of hours per night) ____________________
c) your average sleep efficiency (your average sleep time divided by your average time in bed) ____________________

6. Track your sleep quality and the consistency of your rising time by noting:

   a) your average sleep-quality rating from your sleep diaries ______________________________

   b) the number of days you arose within half an hour of your desired rising time ____________________

7. How often did you practice sleep-scheduling and stimulus-control techniques this week (circle one)?

   regularly

   occasionally

   never

8. How often did you engage in sleep-enhancing lifestyle practices this week (circle one)?

   regularly

   occasionally

   never

9. Check all areas of progress listed below that you have made since beginning this program:

   ______ experiencing fewer insomnia nights

   ______ experiencing more nights of core sleep

   ______ experiencing more nights of good sleep

   ______ falling asleep faster

   ______ waking less often during the night

   ______ waking for shorter periods of time during the night

   ______ averaging more sleep time per night

   ______ improved quality of sleep

   ______ improved sleep efficiency

   ______ decreased sleep medication

10. Summarize any positive changes you have noticed in yourself and your life as a result of this program:

____

____

____

____

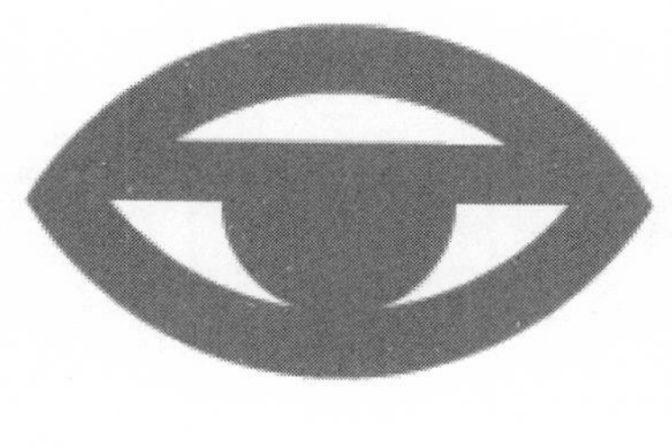

PART III

MANAGING INSOMNIA BY MANAGING STRESS

CHAPTER EIGHT

The Relaxation Response

Imagine a treatment that promotes relaxation and sleep, reduces stress and negative emotions, improves joy and well-being, and facilitates greater control over the body and stress-related health problems such as hypertension, headaches, and pain. This treatment actually exists—and it is safe and costs nothing!

No, it's not a new miracle drug. It's the relaxation response, an inborn, quieting response that is elicited by muscular relaxation, mental focusing, and breathing techniques.

This chapter will explore the stress and relaxation responses and their effects on sleep, emotions, and health. Techniques for eliciting the relaxation response and making it part of your everyday life will also be explored.

On a deeper level, we will look at how the relaxation response can be used to cultivate more inner peace, well-being, and a more profound sense of self.

The Stress Response

To Fight or to Flee

The stress response is a set of involuntary physiological changes that occur whenever we are faced with a threatening or stressful situation. These changes are initiated by an area of the brain called the hypothalamus; they propel the body into a state of arousal and preparation for fighting or fleeing.

The physiological changes of the stress response include:

- Increased amounts of stress hormones such as adrenaline that activate the nervous system and put us "on edge"
- Increased heart rate, blood pressure, and respiration for greater physical strength and energy
- Heightened sensory acuity (improved vision and hearing) and faster brain waves for enhanced alertness and mental reactions
- Decreased blood flow to the stomach and extremities; increased blood flow to the brain, muscles, heart, and lungs to assist in fighting or fleeing
- Increased muscle tension, an evolutionary mechanism that allowed our ancestors to assess danger and remain immobile so they weren't seen by predators; prepare for fight or flight; and create a body armor that provided protection from injury
- Increased sweating to cool the body
- Increased blood-sugar levels to reduce fatigue and increase energy

We have all experienced a frightening event such as a near traffic accident that triggered the stress response: the rush of adrenaline and pounding heart followed by a lightning quick response and a release of energy. Once the danger passed, we heaved a sigh of relief and returned to baseline.

The stress response, also called the fight-or-flight response, is a survival mechanism that was designed to assist our ancestors in fighting or fleeing acute, well-defined physical threats such as predators. Although the response is still useful and necessary, we do not often face the physical stressors of our ancestors. Our personal stressors are more chronic, frequent, and psychological: relationships, work, family, money.

We must also cope with an unprecedented number of social and environmental stressors in a world that transforms itself more rapidly each day:

- Changing social roles, especially for women
- The decline of the nuclear and extended family
- Noise pollution and overcrowding
- Exposure to rapidly increasing amounts of information and global events via computers and mass communications
- Constant sense of time pressure

The brain does not distinguish between physical and psychological stressors. In fact, just imagining a stressful situation can trigger the stress response. This creates a problem: we can't avoid stress, yet we cannot dissipate the physical arousal from the stress response by fighting or fleeing. In the modern-day world with its codes of civilized behavior, fighting and fleeing are not considered acceptable responses to stressful situations. When your boss informs you that you are being fired, you cannot hit him or literally run away from the situation.

The result is chronic, inappropriate, excessive activation of the stress response, which in itself can become a stressor. For many, the stress response occurs so often in daily life that it has become automatic and unconscious.

The Stress-Illness Connection

It is perhaps ironic that the same stress response that was designed to help us survive can now harm us. The notion that excessive, inappropriate stress responses can cause a variety of health problems has gained widespread scientific acceptance. Hundreds of studies have demonstrated that a large number of health problems are stress-related. In fact, most medical textbooks estimate that 50 to 80 percent of all complaints brought to a physician's office are stress-related. These include:

- Muscle problems: chronic tension, headaches, and back pain
- Cardiovascular problems: increased blood pressure and cholesterol, chest pains, irregular heartbeats, anatomical changes in the heart, constriction of coronary blood vessels, and increased risk of cardiovascular disease
- Gastrointestinal problems: irritable bowel syndrome, abdominal pain, colitis, indigestion, constipation, and diarrhea
- Infertility, premenstrual syndrome
- Anxiety, panic attacks, anger, and depression

These stress-related problems can become stressors in their own right, leading to additional stress responses and an unhealthy cycle.

The latest research on stress demonstrates that it can suppress the immune system, which may affect health and disease processes. Additional studies have shown that the following stressors suppress the functioning of the immune system:

- Marital conflict, separation, divorce, and loneliness
- Job loss and unemployment
- Academic examinations
- Death of a loved one
- Caring for a family member with a debilitating illness

Does this mean that all stress is bad? The answer is no; not all stress can or should be avoided. Some stress is positive and an integral part of personal development and daily life: the birth of a child, moving to a new home, a marriage, or a new job. Research also demonstrates that a certain amount of stress enhances performance and motivation. Periods of stress such as a life-threatening illness can even stimulate profound personal transformation, spirituality, or a reordering of life priorities. In short, a life without stress would be a life without challenge, adaptation, and growth.

Stress becomes a problem when it is excessive and chronic. As research consistently documents, we become even more vulnerable to many types of emotional and physical illnesses when we believe we have little or no control over stress.

The Stress Response and Sleep

It is not surprising that excessive activation of the stress response can also disturb sleep. Stressful life events are the most common precipitators of chronic insomnia and most insomniacs (and some good sleepers) have a harder time sleeping on stressful days.

Studies have documented that the more frequent and intense the daytime stressors, the greater the likelihood of sleep difficulties that night. Research has also shown that increased daytime stress is correlated with reduced deep sleep, which results in lighter, more restless sleep. Other research has shed light on why stress disrupts sleep by demonstrating that daytime stress results in increased amounts of stress hormones throughout the day *and* night. In other words, when you are stressed during the day, your stress hormones are not just elevated during the day; they are also elevated while you sleep. Consequently, the wakefulness system is too stimulated, making insomnia more likely.

It is not only daytime stress responses that disturb sleep. As we noted in chapter 5, stress responses are also caused by negative sleep thoughts at bedtime or during the night. These responses play a powerful role in stimulating the wakefulness system and causing insomnia.

In my research, I found that, compared to good sleepers, insomniacs exhibit faster brain waves before and during the early stages of sleep. Other researchers have shown that insomniacs also exhibit faster brain waves during dream sleep. Taken together, these findings suggest that insomniacs have a more difficult time sleeping, in part because their wakefulness system is too stimulated by the stress response.

Fortunately, we have a tool within us that can improve sleep by countering daily stress responses and allowing us to produce the physiological changes associated with sleep: the relaxation response.

The Relaxation Response

Using the Mind to Control the Body

Prior to the 1960s, voluntary control over the autonomic nervous system, or the branch of the body that controls respiration, heart rate, and other "automatic" functions, was considered impossible. In the late 1960s, exciting discoveries in the field of biofeedback challenged this belief.

Biofeedback involves the use of electronic instrumentation to measure physiological information that we are normally unaware of, such as brain waves and heart rate. The information is fed back to the individual using auditory tones or visual signals, thereby giving the person precise information concerning subtle, unconscious physiological processes.

Scientists discovered that, by altering mental activity (thoughts, images, concentration, and attention), and using the biofeedback signal as a "mirror," it is possible to achieve greater control over the autonomic nervous system.

Since the 1960s, hundreds of studies have shown that biofeedback can be used to gain more control over brain waves, heart rate, blood pressure, blood flow, skin temperature, muscle tension, and many other physiological processes. These studies offered the first convincing scientific evidence that the mind can be used to control the body.

Marilyn came to me for biofeedback treatment of Raynaud's disease, which is characterized by painful episodes of cold hands caused by constriction of blood vessels, especially during cold weather.

When she began biofeedback treatment, she was connected to a thermal biofeedback machine that measured her hand temperature and displayed it as a vertical bar on a computer monitor. When Marilyn's hands cooled, the bar fell; when her hands warmed, the bar rose.

Over a series of sessions, Marilyn learned that when she thought about mental images of warmth, her hands became warmer. However, if she tried too hard to warm her hands, they became colder.

Soon she learned to increase the temperature of her hands from 70 to 95 degrees in as little as ten minutes. With practice, she was able to warm her hands without the biofeedback machine. Eventually, she was able to use her mind alone to keep her hands warm and abort a Raynaud's attack.

The results of biofeedback research were so impressive that many scientists began studying other mind-body techniques such as meditation and relaxation, which scientists found could also be used to gain more control over the autonomic nervous system.

My mentor, Dr. Herbert Benson, was one of the earliest scientists to conduct research on biofeedback, meditation, and relaxation techniques. After years of research, Dr. Benson was struck by the fact that these techniques each produced the same physiological quieting response, which he called the relaxation response (RR).

Dr. Benson proposed that the RR is our body's inborn counterbalancing mechanism to the stress response and can be used to offset the harmful effects of the stress response. He defined the physiological changes of the relaxation response:

- Slower brain-wave patterns and mental quieting
- Reduced secretion of stress hormones
- Reductions in heart and breathing rates and, in some cases, blood pressure
- Increased blood flow to the extremities
- Relaxation of the muscles throughout the body

Dr. Benson also defined the four key elements necessary to elicit the RR:

- A quiet place with eyes closed to minimize distractions
- A comfortable position and muscular relaxation
- A mental focusing device such as breathing, a word, or an image to shift the mind away from distracting thoughts
- Passive disregard of everyday thoughts

Although the RR occurs automatically in response to physical stressors, which involve an expenditure of energy, the same does not hold true for psychological stressors. Therefore, we must learn to consciously elicit the RR to counter the effects of excessive stress responses. Later in this chapter you will learn how to elicit the RR.

The Health Benefits of Relaxation

A significant amount of research has demonstrated that the RR is an effective treatment for many health problems, including:

- Anxiety disorders and panic attacks
- Headaches, back pain, arthritis, cancer pain, and other chronic pain conditions
- Gastrointestinal problems such as irritable bowel syndrome
- Hypertension, angina, and heart disease
- Menopausal hot flashes, premenstrual syndrome, and infertility
- Nausea and vomiting due to chemotherapy

The RR is also used to stabilize blood-sugar levels in diabetics and to speed recovery from surgery. It is routinely used to reduce the length of labor and discomfort in childbirth and has been shown to strengthen the immune system and increase defenses against upper respiratory infections.

• • •

When I was a postdoctoral fellow at Children's Hospital in Boston, Emily, a nine-year-old, was referred to me for treatment of headaches. Emily's headaches occurred almost daily and were not responding to medication.

Emily's treatment involved learning to manage headaches by using the RR to control muscle tension in her neck, shoulders, and face.

After one week of practice, Emily reduced the frequency and severity of her headaches by 50 percent. After several more weeks, she cut her headaches to two per week and was no longer taking medication. Eventually, she was able to reduce her headaches to twice per month.

Emily's story demonstrates that the RR can be highly effective in the treatment of headaches and in some cases more effective than medication.

Relaxation and Sleep

Dozens of scientific studies have proven that the RR is an effective treatment for insomnia. The RR improves sleep because, when practiced during the day, it counters daily stress responses, thereby reducing the likelihood that stress hormones will be elevated at night. The RR also improves sleep because, when practiced at bedtime or after an awakening, it helps turn off negative sleep thoughts, quiet the mind, and relax the body.

My research suggests another reason the RR improves sleep: it produces a brain-wave pattern similar to Stage 1 sleep. Recall that Stage 1 is the transition state between waking and sleeping and is characterized by theta brain waves; consequently, by practicing the RR at bedtime or after a nighttime awakening, it is easier to enter Stage 1 sleep and ultimately Stage 2, deep sleep, and dream sleep.

When Tom came to my insomnia program, he regularly awakened during the middle of the night for several hours. Some nights, he never fell back to sleep and slept as little as two hours. Tom's insomnia was more pronounced after stressful days at work. He often lay awake, rehashing the day's events.

As part of Tom's treatment, he practiced the RR at lunchtime and when he woke up in the middle of the night. The first time he used the RR at lunchtime, he found himself entering a pleasant, drowsy state. After just a few nights of practicing the RR after a nighttime wake-up, Tom was able to quiet his mind and fall back to sleep more easily.

Eventually, Tom was able to use the RR on most nights to fall back to sleep within twenty minutes. His sleep time gradually increased to over five hours a night. He felt more rested in the morning and developed a greater sense of control over his mind and sleep.

Tom's story illustrates that, although the RR by itself may not cure insomnia, it has a significant positive effect on sleep for most insomniacs.

Let's take a closer look at how to elicit the RR.

Learning to Elicit the RR

Step 1: Relax the muscles throughout the body. This is accomplished by lying down or sitting comfortably, closing the eyes, then feeling relaxation gradually spread throughout the body. Some people start with the head and feel relaxation spread to the toes; others find it easier to start with the feet. Feelings of relaxation may vary from warmth, heaviness, tingling, or floating to nothing specific.

Step 2: Establish a relaxed breathing pattern. When relaxed or sleeping, we breathe with the abdomen, which relaxes the body because carbon dioxide is expelled and oxygen inhaled efficiently. Under stress, we tend to breathe using short, shallow, regular chest breaths, or we hold our breath. We don't inhale oxygen and exhale carbon dioxide effectively, which stresses the body. Waste products build up in the bloodstream and we feel more anxious.

You can demonstrate abdominal breathing to yourself simply by placing one hand on your stomach and the other on your chest. Without trying to slow or deepen breathing, simply focus on breathing with the abdomen. If you are breathing abdominally, only the hand on your stomach will move. As you breath abdominally, respiration will slow and deepen naturally.

You can demonstrate breath holding to yourself by making a fist in front of your face. Concentrate on creating as much tension in the fist as possible. Hold the tension for about ten seconds, then relax your hand.

What happened to your breathing while you made the fist? You held it! This simple exercise demonstrates that breath holding is so ingrained that it has become an unconscious habit.

Step 3: Direct your attention from everyday thoughts by using a mental focusing device that is neutral and repetitive: a word such as *one, relax, peace,* or *heavy,* or any word you choose; or, the rise and fall of the abdomen as you breathe. For many, it is helpful to repeat a word silently with each exhalation.

The mental focusing device can also be a visual image of an enjoyable, relaxing place:

- A favorite vacation spot
- A place you create
- A beach, a meadow, or mountain
- A place in a book, magazine, or movie
- Floating on a cloud

When eliciting the RR, it is important to assume a passive attitude. In other words, let relaxation happen at its own pace; don't "try" to relax, and don't worry about whether relaxation is occurring. If distracting thoughts occur, disregard them and return attention to the mental focusing device.

Now you understand the three steps in eliciting the RR and are ready to try it. Read the following instructions, then close your eyes and mentally repeat them (you can also record the instructions on a cassette tape and play them back or have someone read them to you):

Sit in a chair or lie on a bed or floor and get comfortable. Close your eyes and direct your attention to the toes and feet. Begin to feel a wave of relaxation move through the feet. (You may notice a sensation of warmth, tingling, or heaviness, or you may just feel your feet against your shoes or the floor.) It may help to visualize relaxation moving through the feet.

Now feel or visualize relaxation moving up through the calves. Next, feel it move up to the thighs, taking time to notice how relaxed the legs are becoming. Now feel the relaxation move up to the stomach, chest, and then over to the back. Your upper body is becoming more and more relaxed.

Feel relaxation moving out to the hands, where again you may notice a sensation of warmth, tingling, or heaviness. Perhaps you feel your hands against the body, chair, or bed. Feel or visualize relaxation moving up to the forearms, upper arms, and shoulders, taking a few moments to concentrate on this. Next, the relaxation moves to the neck, jaw, cheeks, eyes, and forehead.

Relaxation has now moved throughout the entire body, which is becoming more and more relaxed. Take a few moments to concentrate on whole-body relaxation.

Focus your attention now on breathing. Note that it is becoming more rhythmic and abdominal. Also notice that as you inhale, the stomach expands; as you exhale, it contracts. Take a few moments to focus attention on abdominal breathing. It may help to visualize a helium-filled balloon in the abdomen. As you inhale, the balloon fills with air; when you exhale, it gets smaller. If the mind drifts to distracting, everyday thoughts, simply let them go and return attention to breathing.

> You are breathing more rhythmically and abdominally. It may help to pick a word to repeat silently to yourself each time that you exhale. This word will serve as a focus of attention to direct the mind away from distracting, everyday thoughts. Take a few moments to focus on breathing and the word.
>
> Finally, at your own pace, take a slow, deep breath and slowly open your eyes.

What was your experience like? When people first elicit the RR, they often experience physical relaxation: the muscles relax, breathing and heart rate slow. Others notice novel sensations such as heaviness, warmth, tingling, or even floating. Most are amazed, however, to find how difficult it is to quiet the mind, which wanders from thought to thought as if it has a life of its own.

The tendency of the mind to wander during the RR is normal at first. With practice, the ability to quiet the mind and focus attention improves. Thoughts begin to slow and pleasantly drift.

During deep relaxation, you may feel that you are not really awake or asleep. You may begin to lose awareness of surroundings, thoughts, or the mental focusing device and enter a state similar to Stage 1 sleep. If attention drifts back to everyday thoughts, return to the mental focusing device until the mind quiets again.

Initially, feelings of relaxation from the RR may only be temporary. However, in as little as a few weeks, the body's stress hormones become less reactive and the effects of the RR begin to "carry over" and extend throughout the day. As a result, the deleterious effects of stress hormones on sleep are minimized and the following benefits may begin to occur:

- Increased awareness of tension, decreased stress reactions, and a greater ability to produce relaxation quickly and automatically
- Decreased anxiety, anger, frustration, and stress-related symptoms, and improved daytime mood
- Increased sense of control over stress; this, as we have explored, is vital to health and well-being

Some of the beneficial effects of the RR are immediate and obvious; others occur over longer periods of time and are more subtle. Awareness of the benefits of the RR may come from others who comment that your "fuse is not as short." You may recognize the benefits by comparing past stress reactions to present ones.

Guidelines for Establishing Daytime RR Practice

The more consistently the RR is practiced, the greater the benefits for sleep, health, and daily life. The RR needs to be practiced almost daily to obtain significant benefits. If you miss a day or two a week, don't become alarmed, but remember: practicing only a few times per week is usually not sufficient to counter the daily effects of stress on the mind and body.

The most difficult part of establishing regular RR practice is finding time. In our society, many feel the day is too busy for relaxation or feel guilty and unproductive if time for relaxation is taken.

You are more likely to allot time for the RR regularly if you think of it as something that will improve mood, performance, and health; that is as important as eating and exercising appropriately; and that you need and deserve. Ultimately, think of finding time for the RR this way: if you can't find time for it, you are probably one of those most in need of it.

Additional guidelines to realize the many potential benefits of the RR:

1. Allot ten to twenty minutes per day for the RR. Most people simply can't relax and quiet the mind in less time. As more experience is gained, relaxation occurs more quickly. If it is difficult to find twenty minutes during the day, start with ten minutes—but start!

2. Practice the RR in a comfortable position and in a quiet place where you will not be disturbed by noises, telephones, children, pets, and so on. Most people practice the RR at home but it can also be done in a library, conference room, or office. If practiced in the same place regularly, the RR is more likely to become associated with that room and therefore become a habit.

3. Experiment to find the time of day that works best for RR practice, then designate that time as regular RR time. By practicing at the same time each day, the RR will become more habitual. Some find it helpful to start the day with the RR; others find that practicing later in the day, when stress responses have accumulated, is more effective.

Recall from our exploration of napping that nature intended an afternoon rest period. Consider afternoon RR practice; it may satisfy the biological tendency for a midafternoon nap or rest. You may even fall asleep during the RR, which is fine—you will learn to associate the RR with sleep. Be careful about eliciting the RR within an hour or two of bedtime because you may fall asleep in the form of a short nap and therefore have a harder time doing so at bedtime.

4. Additional RR scripts can be found in appendix D. Experiment and find those you like. After almost twenty years of teaching patients the RR, I find the most effective way to learn it is by using an RR cassette tape. A tape makes it easier to focus attention and keep the mind from wandering. Consider making a tape of the RR scripts in this book, or purchase an RR tape at one of the many bookstores that sell them. The RR tape that I recorded and use with my patients can be ordered using the information in the back of this book (see p. 216).

5. A small percentage of patients do not seem to relax effectively using the RR. If, after a few weeks of practice, you do not experience relaxation or perhaps feel agitated during the RR, discontinue its practice and focus on the other techniques in this program.

Using the RR to Induce Sleep

During the first few days of RR practice, do not use it to fall asleep at bedtime or after a nighttime wake-up. Why? Because you may try too hard to relax and become frustrated. Wait until you have practiced the RR during the day often enough that you are relaxing consistently (this may take a few days or even a week), then begin using it to induce sleep after lights out or if you awaken during the night and don't quickly fall back to sleep. If you are using a cassette for daytime practice, the sound of the tape recorder turning off may disrupt sleep, a problem that can be avoided by mentally practicing the RR to induce sleep.

With practice, greater consistency develops in using the RR to fall asleep. Consequently, it will become associated with sleep and your sense of control over sleep will be enhanced.

Be realistic; don't expect the RR to induce sleep every night. If you elicit the RR and don't fall asleep or back to sleep within twenty to thirty minutes, follow the stimulus-control guidelines from the previous chapter: sit up in bed or get out of bed and engage in a relaxing activity until drowsy, then return to bed and try the RR again. Repeat this process until asleep.

If, after a few weeks of practice, the RR does not seem to induce sleep, discontinue its practice in bed. Otherwise, the RR may become associated with frustration.

Minis

How can you elicit the relaxation response in situations with only a few minutes (or seconds) to relax and when the eyes cannot be closed? Examples include:

- At a stop light or in a traffic jam
- During an argument
- Waiting in line
- Just before giving a speech
- Walking into a crowded room

The answer: a mini relaxation—an abbreviated version of the RR. A mini involves taking a few moments to relax the muscles in the body (particularly the neck, shoulders, and face), then practicing abdominal breathing and mental-focusing techniques. A mini can be practiced with the eyes open or closed, sitting or standing, for a few seconds or minutes.

Take a moment now to try a mini. Begin by closing the eyes and taking a few moments to relax the legs, arms, upper body, and face. Next, focus on abdominal breathing for a minute or two. With each exhalation, you may want to mentally focus on a word. If the mind wanders to distracting thoughts, let them go and return attention to the breathing and word. Now open your eyes.

That's all there is to a mini!

Minis may not be as effective as the RR in terms of producing deep relaxation. However, they offer two advantages. First, they can be used anytime, anywhere, to cope with stressful situations as they occur. You will discover that it is possible to perform a mini while in the presence of others or engaged in a conversation and no one will know that you are doing so! Second, minis can be used more frequently than the RR and may therefore be more effective than practicing the RR only once a day.

Carol suffered from anxiety and panic attacks. At times, the attacks were so severe that they prevented her from leaving the house. As part of Carol's treatment, she first learned to elicit the RR once a day. Later, she began to practice minis throughout the day and whenever she felt anxious or noticed the beginning of a panic attack.

After several weeks of using the RR and minis, Carol noticed a reduction in her anxiety and was able to avert many panic attacks by using minis. Although her anxiety wasn't entirely gone, she felt more empowered and in control.

Practicing a mini is easy; remembering to practice one is difficult. There are numerous occasions when we simply don't recognize tension and forget to practice a mini. Therefore, it is necessary to use cues to increase the use of minis. An effective reminder is a small piece of colored tape placed on the crystal of a watch. Each time you glance at the watch, the tape will act as a cue to practice a mini. Other cues are stoplights, television commercials, waiting in line, being on hold on the telephone, and waiting rooms. A sticker on the telephone or reminders taped to the refrigerator or bathroom mirror are good cues; by using them, you will make minis an automatic occurrence when tension is experienced.

Practice minis regularly, for they can improve awareness of subtle levels of tension, distract attention from stressful thoughts, and keep attention focused in the present. They also make the RR more automatic.

The Deeper Benefits of the RR and Minis

Besides reducing stress and improving relaxation and sleep, continued regular practice of the RR and minis can result in the following changes:

1. The RR and minis quiet and clear the mind and improve the ability to focus and concentrate. Consequently, your performance and problem solving may improve.

2. Daily consciousness consists of a constant internal self-dialogue, an endless flood of mental conversation that wanders continuously from the past to the future, hopes and fears, fantasies and desires, arguments and schemes. This internal dialogue dominates our thinking and, as we will explore in the next chapter, plays an important role in causing moods and feelings.

Between the internal dialogue and the hectic daily world, in which we are bombarded by an overload of stressful stimuli, awareness of a sense of inner quiet and calm is often elusive. When the mind is quieted during the RR and minis, a sense of clarity, stillness, and inner peace may be experienced. Over time, this heightened sense of inner peace can begin to extend throughout the day and provide a calmer, more positive outlook on life.

3. Many Eastern traditions emphasize that the internal dialogue has come to occupy so large a place in our consciousness that we regard it as the only state of consciousness, as our sense of self. Self-consciousness is characterized by a tendency to create personal boundaries and perceive the world as "me/not me" and "self/not self"; a tendency to perceive differences, separation, and isolation between self and others; judgment, self-criticism, doubt, fear, frustration, and anxiety.

Using the RR and minis to turn off the internal dialogue will cause a change in perception of one's sense of self. This new sense of self is often described as stronger, more connected, and higher; more selfless and able to perceive similarities and unity between the self and others; more unified, harmonious, integrated, and whole.

This change in self-awareness can foster greater self-esteem and acceptance, inner strength, and a healthier outlook on life. Thus, the RR and minis can be tools for personal transformation and growth.

4. Just as the internal dialogue affects our internal sense of self, it also affects our perceptions of the external world. We navigate on autopilot and tune out many positive aspects of the daily world. We drive to work and don't notice a magnificent sunrise or the beauty of the leaves changing color on a sunny fall day. We are too preoccupied with our own thoughts to hear what is being said, to see what is really in front of us, to "be" in the moment. Some Eastern traditions describe this daily mode of consciousness as a state of "half-sleep."

When the RR and minis are used to quiet our internal dialogue, a shift in awareness of the external world occurs. We become conscious of things that are normally unconscious. We are more likely to hear the meaning in what is being said, really see what is around us, and become more aware of body language and nonverbal communication.

Our attention becomes more fully absorbed in the present, which is more peaceful than worrying about the past and the future. The world is experienced more directly and vividly—the color of a sunset, a smile, the sound of music—as if the senses were cleansed. We see the world more as children do: through a state of absorbed attention, of being rather than thinking. Everyday moments take on a more immediate sense of joy, pleasure, and meaning; life appears more vibrant, less routine and automated.

Recall situations when your attention was completely absorbed in something: bonding with a newborn, lovemaking, a star-filled sky, a beautiful sunrise or sunset, a panoramic view of the ocean, the stillness of the mountains, the sound or sight of a crackling wood fire. Time seems suspended, mental chatter stops, and the mind is clear and focused. Just as these moments of absorbed attention elicit the RR, the RR and minis can be powerful tools for bringing about states of absorbed attention, deepened inner peace, and well-being.

Try the RR and minis and see for yourself. They are powerful mind-body tools for improving your sleep and life.

The Week Four Progress Summary

Your Week Four Progress Summary is included at the end of this chapter. Similar to the Week Three summary, it contains items for tracking the sleep pattern and use of sleep medication, areas of improvement in sleep, use of cognitive-restructuring, sleep-scheduling and stimulus-control techniques, and use of sleep- and health-enhancing lifestyle practices.

The Week Four summary also contains two new items: one for tracking use of the RR and minis, the other for tracking use of the RR to induce sleep.

The summary should be completed after reviewing the seven daily sleep diaries. Then, compare it to the previous weeks' summaries to identify improvements in sleep. Remember, the degree of improvement is directly related to how consistently the techniques in this program are used.

Like the Week Three summary, Week Four contains a section for listing positive changes in other elements of life that occur as a result of this program. In this section, include improvements in life that are experienced as a result of practicing the RR and minis such as:

- Improved ability to recognize and turn off stress responses
- Greater feelings of control over stress; reduction in stress-related symptoms
- Improved concentration and attention
- Enhanced feelings of inner peace and well-being

Now that you have finished the fourth week of this six-week program, it is appropriate to add a new cognitive-restructuring technique. Recall from chapter 5 that the goal of cognitive restructuring is to improve sleep by promoting positive sleep thoughts (PSTs) and minimizing negative sleep thoughts (NSTs). Since the first week of the program, you have been practicing cognitive restructuring by recording your NSTs and PSTs on your daily 60-Second Sleep Diary.

The new cognitive-restructuring technique is designed to reinforce, on a daily basis, the improvements you have made in sleep. To do so, take a moment to look at the sleep diary at the end of this chapter. Notice that it contains an additional item for recording areas of improvement in sleep. When you complete this item each morning, make a notation of at least one of the areas of improvement that you checked off on the weekly progress summary.

Recording sleep improvements in the diary will reinforce the improvements each day and promote PSTs, minimize NSTs, and help you begin every day empowered in the knowledge that you are making positive changes in sleep.

WEEK FOUR PROGRESS SUMMARY

1. Assess your sleep pattern this week by noting:

a) the number of good nights of sleep ________________

b) the number of nights of core sleep (five and a half hours or more) ________________

c) the number of insomnia nights ________________

2. On how many daily sleep diaries did you record a positive sleep thought? ________________

3. How often did you mentally practice cognitive restructuring this week (circle one)?

regularly

occasionally

never

4. Assess your sleep-medication use this week by noting:

a) the number of medication-free nights ________________

b) the number of reduced-dosage nights ________________

c) the number of usual-dosage nights ________________

5. Track your sleep efficiency by calculating:

a) your average sleep time (number of hours per night) ________________

b) your average time in bed (number of hours per night) ________________

c) your average sleep efficiency (your average sleep time divided by your average time in bed) ________________

6. Track your sleep quality and the consistency of your rising time by noting:

a) your average sleep-quality rating from your sleep diaries ______________________________

b) the number of days you arose within half an hour of your desired rising time______________________________

7. How often did you practice sleep-scheduling and stimulus-control techniques this week (circle one)?

regularly

occasionally

never

8. How often did you engage in sleep-enhancing lifestyle practices this week (circle one)?

regularly

occasionally

never

9. How often did you practice the relaxation response and minis during the day (circle one)?

regularly

occasionally

never

10. How often did you practice the relaxation response to help yourself fall asleep or back to sleep at night (circle one)?

regularly

occasionally

never

11. Check all areas of progress listed below that you have made since beginning this program:

______ experiencing fewer insomnia nights

______ experiencing more nights of core sleep

______ experiencing more nights of good sleep

______ falling asleep faster

______ waking less often during the night

______ waking for shorter periods of time during the night

______ averaging more sleep time per night

______ improved quality of sleep

______ improved sleep efficiency

______ decreased sleep medication

12. Summarize any positive changes you have noticed in yourself and your life as a result of this program:

____

____

____

____

60-SECOND SLEEP DIARY

Night ________________ Date ________________

1. Last night, what time did you get into bed? ________________
   Turn the lights off? ________________
2. About how long did it take you to fall asleep? ________________
   ____
3. About how many times did you awaken during the night? _____
   ____
4. For each awakening, about how long were you awake? ________
   1st ________________ 2nd ________________
   3rd ________________ 4th ________________
5. What time was your final wake-up this morning? ____________
   What time did you get out of bed? ________________
6. Approximately how many hours did you sleep last night? ______
   ____
7. How many hours did you allot for sleep last night (time elapsed from "lights out" to "out of bed")? ________________
8. Rate the quality of last night's sleep:

1	2	3	4	5
excellent				poor

9. Sleep medications taken ________________

10. a) NSTs ________________
   b) PSTs ________________

11. Areas of improvement in sleep: ________________
   ____

CHAPTER NINE

Learning to Think Away Your Stress

Kurt had been employed with his company for over three years. He loved his management job and had recently received a superior performance review. Yet, with only two weeks notice, he was told his company was downsizing and that his position was being eliminated.

In the blink of an eye, Kurt's outlook went from rosy to a state of panic. All he could think about was losing his job:

> **"What did I do to deserve this?"**
> **"My luck is always bad."**
> **"I'll never find a good job like this one again."**
> **"I won't be able to pay my rent and will have to move back home with my parents."**
> **"I'll have to postpone my wedding."**

Kurt became more anxious and depressed. He couldn't concentrate or motivate himself. He slept poorly and developed daily headaches.

After a month of being unemployed, feeling depressed, anxious, and not sleeping, Kurt finally put his resume together and started looking for a job. To his surprise, he landed interviews with two companies and received job offers from both. The position he accepted included a 15 percent pay increase over his previous job and a company car.

Kurt was promoted six months later and received a raise. Today he is a rising star with the same company.

As Kurt's story illustrates, it's not just external events that cause our stress and moods; mental reactions also play an important role.

We have all experienced situations that appeared overwhelming at first but later turned out to be much less serious—and sometimes positive. In looking back, we realize that our initial thoughts were overly negative and out of proportion to the situation.

In the preceding chapter, we explored the body's stress response, its adverse effects on sleep and health, and how to counter these effects using the relaxation response. In this chapter, we will build on this foundation and explore yet another method for managing stress: cognitive restructuring, which in this case means to change our mental responses to stress.

In chapter 5 we examined how negative sleep thoughts cause stress responses that trigger insomnia, and the use of cognitive restructuring to minimize negative sleep thoughts, promote positive sleep thoughts, and improve sleep.

Similarly, cognitive restructuring for stress management is based on the idea that we often respond to daily stressful events with negative, distorted thoughts. These thoughts create negative emotions, trigger the stress response, and ultimately disturb sleep, health, and well-being.

Just as cognitive restructuring can be used to manage negative sleep thoughts, it can be used to control negative thoughts and emotions about daily stressors. Consequently, stress responses and stress-related health problems can be reduced, and the likelihood that stress responses will cause stress hormones to stay elevated at night and disturb sleep can be minimized.

Combining cognitive restructuring and the relaxation response provides a highly effective approach to reducing the impact of daily stress on sleep, health, and life: cognitive restructuring for managing the thoughts that lead to emotional stress and the relaxation response for countering the body's physical responses to stress.

Stress and Negative Self-Talk

We constantly talk to ourselves about events in our daily lives, describing what is happening, going to happen, and should happen, why things happen, and so on. This self-talk is continual, automatic, and occurs partially outside of awareness. Consequently, we don't pay much attention to it or realize that when faced with stressful situations our self-talk changes in distinct ways.

First, our mind assumes "tunnel vision," focusing on the stressful event and becoming preoccupied with it—for example, when Kurt lost his job, he could not think about anything else. Second, the mind becomes a negative filter. Dr. David Burns, of the Presbyterian Medical Center of Philadelphia and a pioneer in cognitive-restructuring techniques, likens this filter to a strong pair of eyeglasses that distorts our view of the world. The filter allows in only negative, distorted thoughts, called negative automatic thoughts, or NATs.

For example, if you get a message that your boss would like to see you immediately, your NATs might be:

"Oh, no, not again!"
"What did I do wrong?"
"What now?"
"Am I going to lose my job?"

For someone who has to take a major exam, NATs might be:

"I'm dreading this."
"What if I fail?"
"I won't be prepared."

NATs are like knee-jerk reactions to stress that occur almost unconsciously, automatically, and without any effort. They typically involve worst-case scenarios, jumping to conclusions, "awfulizing," and "catastrophizing." They seem so real that we don't stop to question or examine them, and we believe them as if they were facts or absolute truths. Consequently, NATs cause us to lose perspective, get locked into one-track thinking, accentuate the negative, and view stressful situations in an inaccurate, distorted fashion.

Because NATs are stressful and overpowering, they take precedence in our thinking. Thus, we forget positive events easily and have a more difficult time ridding stressful events from our minds. The more repetitive and constant NATs become, the more they occur in the back of our minds, making it more difficult to catch and examine them, and to prevent them from triggering negative emotions and stress responses.

Why does the mind assume tunnel vision, become a negative filter, and let in only NATs under stress? Recent research by Dr. Joseph Ledoux of New York University suggests that these mental responses to stress may be a consequence of survival mechanisms that assisted our ancestors in dealing with physical stressors such as predators.

According to Ledoux, our ancestors were more likely to survive physical threats if, one, their thoughts narrowed, assumed tunnel vision, and focused solely on the threat at hand without distraction; and two, they responded quickly and automatically, almost unconsciously, to stressors without much conscious deliberation. Thus, if they heard a rustle in the bushes, it was advantageous to quickly and automatically interpret the rustle as a predator because it may have meant the difference between life and death.

Ledoux points out that these reactions to stress are so rapid and reflexive that they sacrifice accuracy for speed and therefore increase the likelihood of "false alarms." For instance, the rustle in the bushes may in fact have been only the wind. However, from an evolutionary perspective, it is better to be safe and overreact than underact and be sorry—or dead.

These mental responses to stress, once necessary for survival, are no longer as adaptive for today's frequent, excessive psychological stressors that don't involve physical danger and survival. The mind's tunnel vision and false alarms under stress create a negative filter that triggers NATs, which cause excessive, unnecessary, negative emotions such as anxiety, fear, or anger. These emotions, which can become stressors in their own right, elicit stress responses that affect our mood and health and increase the likelihood that stress hormones will disturb sleep.

Reframing Negative Self-Talk

Some negative thoughts and emotions are normal responses to stressful situations, such as grieving after a death. These negative emotions are usually time-limited and occur in response to stressors that would trigger similar feelings in most people. Negative emotions can also be adaptive, for they motivate us to change, grow, overcome obstacles, and achieve goals.

For many people, however, negative emotions such as anxiety, frustration, and anger are excessive, unhealthy, and trigger excessive stress responses that adversely affect sleep, thinking, motivation, and health. We often can't change the situations that cause stress, but we can change our emotional responses to stress using cognitive restructuring. This technique involves learning to recognize and change NATs so that we can:

- Be more realistic and accurate in thinking about stressful situations
- Reduce tunnel vision under stress
- See stressful situations more clearly
- Minimize "false alarms" in response to stressors

Consequently, cognitive restructuring can help us to achieve greater control over negative emotions and stress responses. Our mood and health improve, stress hormones are not as likely to remain elevated at night, and sleep improves.

Let's take a closer look at how to practice cognitive restructuring for stress management.

Recognizing NATs

The first step in cognitive restructuring is to become more aware of NATs. Many people have difficulty with this step because NATs are so automatic. The most effective way to recognize NATs is to track them in writing. This will allow you to become aware of how often you engage in NATs, objectively examine and weigh them, and see how distorted and inaccurate they are.

Take a moment to look at the Cognitive Restructuring Diary at the end of this chapter. Each day, choose one or two stressful situations that triggered negative emotions and briefly describe the situations in the column labeled "Situation." Next, record the NATs that filtered through your mind before and during the stressful situation in the column labeled "NATs." Ask yourself, "What were my negative thoughts and what was I saying to myself about the situation that contributed to my feelings of stress?"

Neil was a forty-five-year-old advertising professional who wanted to reduce excessive anxiety, anger, and stress-related symptoms such as insomnia, headaches, and muscle tension. As part of his stress-management training, Neil learned about his NATs and their effect on his emotions and health. He then practiced the first step in cognitive restructuring: recognizing NATs by tracking them on paper.

After one week of recording his NATs using the Cognitive Restructuring Diary, Neil was able to identify several situations each day in which his NATs triggered anxiety or anger. For example, when driving to work his NATs were:

"That jerk cut me off; who the heck does he think he is?"
"Oh no, a traffic jam; I'll be late for the meeting."
"Why do I hit every red stop light?"
"This traffic drives me crazy!"

Before a major presentation for a client, Neil's NATs were:

> **"I'm too nervous to do a good job."**
> **"I probably won't get the account."**
> **"I won't be prepared."**
> **"I bet they won't like my presentation."**

Neil found that noting his NATs on the Cognitive Restructuring Diary was one of the most helpful things he had ever done for understanding his emotional responses to stress. He had never realized how frequently he engaged in NATs or how negative and automatic they were.

Three Methods for Reframing NATs

After learning to become aware of NATs using the Cognitive Restructuring Diary, the next step is to reframe them by writing down more accurate, adaptive thoughts about stressful situations. The third column of the diary, labeled "Reframed Thought," is used for this purpose.

Reframing NATs is not always easy. Fortunately, there are a number of proven techniques that will make this step easier.

First, ask yourself the following ten key questions:

1. Is this thought really true?
2. Am I overemphasizing a negative aspect of this situation?
3. What is the worst thing that will happen?
4. Is there anything that might be positive about this situation?
5. Am I "catastrophizing," "awfulizing," jumping to conclusions, and assuming a negative outcome?
6. How do I know this situation will turn out this way?
7. Is there another way to look at this situation?
8. What difference will this make next week, month, or year?

9. If I had one month to live, how important would this be?
10. Am I using words such as *never, always, worst, terrible*, or *horrible* to describe the situation?

These ten key reframing questions are critical for they will help you see the inaccuracies and distortions in your NATs; view each NAT not as a fact but as only one of many ways of looking at a stressful situation; and substitute more realistic, accurate thoughts about stressful situations.

Second, use the "double standard" technique developed by Dr. Burns. This technique is based on the idea that, when it comes to explaining stressful events, we are often much harder on ourselves than we are on our friends. We operate on a double standard: we have realistic and fair standards that we apply to others whom we care about, yet we encourage them to reframe their reactions to stressful events. In contrast, we set unrealistic standards for ourselves when we explain stressful events to ourselves.

To use the double-standard technique, examine your NATs and ask yourself: "Would I say this to a close friend with a similar problem? If not, what would I say to him or her?" Reframe your NATs by giving yourself the same encouraging messages you would give a friend.

Third, reflect on past experience and ask yourself, "Has anything like this happened to me in the past and, if so, how did it turn out?" By doing so, we can often prove to ourselves that many of the things we worry about never happen, or don't turn out as badly as we have imagined.

Kayla, an actress and insomniac, had just finished a play and received a standing ovation. At a reception afterwards, her friends and family offered her congratulations and praise on her performance. "This was your best performance ever!" said one friend. "Incredible!" said another.

One friend, however, suggested that Kayla could have done better during one scene. Instantly, Kayla's entire perception of her performance changed. Her NATs were:

"I didn't do as good a job as I thought."
"Will I ever be a good actress?"
"What other scenes did I mess up?"
"The review in tomorrow's paper won't be positive."

When Kayla got home, she noted her NATs on the Cognitive Restructuring Diary. Just by seeing them in writing, she began to see how negative they were. Kayla then used the ten key reframing questions and wrote down these reframed thoughts in her diary:

"I overemphasized one comment from one person."
"I jumped to conclusions; even if one scene wasn't great, that doesn't mean my other scenes were not good."
"I couldn't have performed poorly; I received a standing ovation."
"No performance is perfect."

Kayla also reframed her NATs by using a past experience; she recalled the time she thought she had given an average performance yet received a good review in the newspaper.

By reframing her NATs, Kayla felt better. She went to bed that night focusing on the positive aspects of her performance and slept well. Best of all, she woke up to a great review of the performance in the local paper. She was thrilled and couldn't wait until her next performance.

The Stop-Mini-Reframe Technique

Once you gain experience recognizing and reframing NATs using the Cognitive Restructuring Diary, you are ready for the final step in cognitive restructuring: recognizing and reframing NATs as they filter through your mind. The following technique, called the Stop-Mini-Reframe technique, is a highly effective method that will help you implement this final step:

1. *Stop:* When encountering a stressful situation, say "Stop" to yourself before your NATs escalate. Simply saying "Stop" can help you break the cycle of NATs, negative emotions, and stress responses.
2. *Mini:* After you say "Stop" to yourself, practice a mini by relaxing your muscles and focusing on abdominal breathing. This will relax you, divert your attention away from NATs, and help break the cycle of NATs and negative emotions.
3. *Reframe:* Once you have practiced a mini, reframe your NATs using one of the three reframing techniques: the ten key reframing questions, the double-standard technique, reflection on past experience.

Ali is waiting to give her first paper presentation at a scientific conference. Her hands are sweaty, her heart is pounding, and her stomach is in a knot. Her mind is racing with these NATs:

"I have never spoken in front of hundreds of people before!"
"What if I can't answer their questions?"
"What if I talk too fast?"
"I feel like I'm going to faint."
"I'm not as good a speaker as these other people."

Fortunately, Ali knew the Stop-Mini-Reframe technique. She told herself to stop and practiced a mini. Immediately, she felt more relaxed. Then Ali reframed her NATs by using the ten key reframing questions to tell herself:

"I know this material better than anyone."
"Some stress is good—it will help my performance."
"I'm well prepared for this talk."
"I will relax as I begin my talk."

Ali's palms were still sweaty, but she felt much less anxious. When it was her turn to speak, she walked up to the podium, took a few deep breaths, then began her talk. To her surprise, she spoke slowly and confidently, gave a strong presentation, and handled the audience's questions effectively. She also received a loud round of applause.

Afterwards, Ali felt euphoric. She had spoken well and given a great presentation.

Because NATs are so automatic and habitual, the Stop-Mini-Reframe technique takes some time to learn. But, with practice, you, too, can learn to use Stop-Mini-Reframe anytime, anywhere to:

- Turn off the negative stress filter
- Catch and reframe NATs
- Control negative emotions, stress responses, and stress-related health problems
- Heighten feelings of relaxation and control over stress

These benefits will minimize the adverse effects of stress on sleep. Your mood, energy, and ability to think positively will also improve, which will have a positive effect on your relationships, job performance, and outlook on life. You will also realize the powerful effect your thoughts have on your emotions and well-being.

Cognitive Restructuring and the Relaxation Response: A Powerful Combination

Now you have two highly effective stress-reduction techniques: cognitive restructuring and the relaxation response. The more consistently you practice these techniques, the greater your ability to control the impact of stress on sleep, health, and life.

You can use cognitive restructuring and the relaxation response on nights when NATs about daytime stressors are keeping you awake: cognitive restructuring to reframe NATs and the relaxation response to relax the mind and body. Some find it helpful to use both techniques in combination; others find that one technique works well. Experiment and find the approach that works for you.

If, after using cognitive restructuring and the relaxation response, you still are not asleep within twenty to thirty minutes, follow the stimulus-control guidelines that we have explored: sit up in bed or get out of bed and engage in a relaxing activity until drowsy, then return to bed and use cognitive restructuring and the relaxation response again. Repeat this process until you fall asleep.

Finally, when you get into bed at night, or if you awaken during the night, you will fall asleep more easily if you get in the habit of focusing on positive thoughts in general. Examples:

- Something positive in your life
- An accomplishment or pleasurable experience from the day
- Something you are looking forward to
- Your most enjoyable vacation

Positive thoughts like these distract you from NATs, produce positive emotions, and make it easier to elicit the RR and fall asleep.

The Week Five Progress Summary

A Week Five Progress Summary is included at the end of this chapter. It is similar to the Week Four summary, with one exception: a new item for tracking use of cognitive-restructuring techniques for stress management. In the section for summarizing positive life changes that occur as a result of this program, make notations of improvements experienced as a result of practicing cognitive restructuring for stress management such as:

- Improved ability to recognize and reframe negative thoughts and think more positively
- Improved ability to control negative emotions, stress responses, and stress-related symptoms

- Enhanced feelings of relaxation, peace of mind, and well-being

Reinforcing these positive changes will enhance self-esteem and confidence. You will also view yourself in a more powerful way and develop a greater sense of control over your life.

COGNITIVE RESTRUCTURING DIARY

Situation	NATs	Reframed Thought

WEEK FIVE PROGRESS SUMMARY

1. Assess your sleep pattern this week by noting:
a) the number of good nights of sleep ______________________
b) the number of nights of core sleep (five and a half hours or more) ______________________
c) the number of insomnia nights ______________________

2. On how many daily sleep diaries did you record a positive sleep thought? ______________________

3. How often did you mentally practice cognitive restructuring for negative sleep thoughts this week (circle one)?
regularly
occasionally
never

4. Assess your sleep-medication use this week by noting:
a) the number of medication-free nights ______________________
b) the number of reduced-dosage nights ______________________
c) the number of usual-dosage nights ______________________

5. Track your sleep efficiency by calculating:
a) your average sleep time (number of hours per night) ______________________
b) your average time in bed (number of hours per night) ______________________
c) your average sleep efficiency (your average sleep time divided by your average time in bed) ______________________

6. Track your sleep quality and the consistency of your rising time by noting:
   a) your average sleep-quality rating from your sleep diaries ______________________________
   b) the number of days you arose within half an hour of your desired rising time ______________________________

7. How often did you practice sleep-scheduling and stimulus-control techniques this week (circle one)?
   regularly
   occasionally
   never

8. How often did you engage in sleep-enhancing lifestyle practices this week (circle one)?
   regularly
   occasionally
   never

9. How often did you practice the relaxation response and minis during the day (circle one)?
   regularly
   occasionally
   never

10. How often did you practice the relaxation response to help yourself fall asleep or back to sleep at night (circle one)?
   regularly
   occasionally
   never

11. How often did you practice cognitive restructuring for stress management this week (circle one)?

regularly

occasionally

never

12. Check all areas of progress listed below that you have made since beginning this program:

______ experiencing fewer insomnia nights

______ experiencing more nights of core sleep

______ experiencing more nights of good sleep

______ falling asleep faster

______ waking less often during the night

______ waking for shorter periods of time during the night

______ averaging more sleep time per night

______ improved quality of sleep

______ improved sleep efficiency

______ decreased sleep medication

13. Summarize any positive changes you have noticed in yourself and your life as a result of this program:

____

____

____

____

CHAPTER TEN

Developing Stress-Reducing, Sleep-Enhancing Attitudes and Beliefs

Ever wonder why some people cope effectively, stay healthy, and sleep well under stress while others don't? The answer, in part, is that individuals who manage stress effectively have developed a constellation of attitudes and beliefs that are stress-reducing.

Take Jim and Kevin for example. When faced with stressful situations, Jim responds by thinking negatively and feeling threatened, feeling helpless and withdrawing from people, and getting angry and losing his sense of humor.

In contrast, Kevin responds by thinking optimistically and viewing stress as a challenge, believing that he can exert some control over stress, laughing at himself and reframing angry thoughts, and seeking out friends and family.

Consequently, Jim feels anxious, experiences headaches, and sleeps poorly under stress. Kevin maintains a positive mood and sleeps well under stress.

The latest research on the mind and health suggests that Kevin's stress-resistant attitudes and beliefs are vital to health and well-being and may extend life.

In preceding chapters, we explored two methods for managing the deleterious effects of stress on mood, sleep, and health: the relaxation response and cognitive restructuring. This chapter will introduce a third technique for managing stress: stress-resistant attitudes and beliefs.

Like the relaxation response and cognitive restructuring, stress-resistant attitudes and beliefs can contribute to more joy, peace of mind, and a healthier outlook on life. By combining these attitudes and beliefs with the relaxation response and cognitive restructuring, you will develop a powerful three-pronged approach to minimizing the adverse effects of stress on sleep, health, and well-being.

The Benefits of Optimism

Optimists are people who focus on and expect positive experiences. They are more likely to attribute positive outcomes to themselves and believe they can influence events through their actions. Optimists also expect the best when faced with uncertainty, look on the bright side, are positive about the future, count on good things to happen, and remember success better than failure. In short, optimists see the silver lining in every cloud.

While optimists certainly experience some negative thoughts and emotions, their positive attitudes and beliefs create a mental filter that allows in primarily positive thoughts while preventing negative ones. Therefore, optimists do not experience a lot of negative thoughts, can change from negative to positive thinking easily, and experience a more positive mood and greater self-esteem and well-being than pessimists.

Studies document that optimism improves health, reduces susceptibility to disease, and may increase life expectancy. One study found that a pessimistic personality style predicted which college students would report more sick days and visits to a physician. In another study, which involved members of the Harvard University classes of 1939 through 1944, men were rated on levels of optimism and pessimism at age twenty-five, then tracked for thirty years. Overall, the men who were pessimistic at age twenty-five were less healthy and had more chronic illness later in life than the men who were optimistic.

Other studies show that optimistic people recover faster from surgery, have fewer medical complications during and after surgery, and exhibit stronger measures of immune functioning than pessimists.

Although optimism may be due in part to inborn temperament, it can be learned. The two stress-reduction methods we have previously explored, cognitive restructuring and the relaxation response, promote optimistic thinking by reducing negative thoughts, emotions, and stress responses, and by increasing one's sense of control over stress.

Here are some additional strategies for promoting optimistic thoughts, attitudes, and beliefs:

1. View setbacks as temporary. If you receive a poor grade on an exam, don't take the attitude that you will perform poorly on subsequent exams. Similarly, a job interview that doesn't lead to an offer should not create the belief that you will never land a job.
2. Avoid generalizing a problem to your whole life. If a relationship doesn't work out, don't tell yourself that your relationships always turn sour. If you throw a party that is a flop, don't tell yourself "I mess up everything."
3. Refrain from dismissing positive events as temporary or due to luck or external causes. If things go well the first month on a new job, don't say "This is beginner's luck that won't last."
4. As advised in the following quote by the late Reinhold Niebuhr, an American theologian, avoid blaming yourself for things beyond your control. "God grant me the serenity to accept the things I cannot change, the courage to change the things I can, and the wisdom to know the difference."
5. Use optimistic affirmations—positive beliefs that are repeated to yourself regularly. An example: "I expect the best when faced with uncertainty." Repeat optimistic affirmations to yourself while taking a morning shower, when practicing the relaxation response, while driving the car, or before going to sleep. Over time, these affirmations will become more automatic than pessimistic beliefs.

6. Practice an "attitude of gratitude." Focus on what you have and on positive events in daily life.
7. Seek out optimists and avoid pessimists. Optimism and pessimism are contagious.

Practice these techniques for developing optimistic thinking. They will minimize negative thoughts, emotions, and stress responses, and improve mood, sleep, and health.

The Three Cs: Control, Commitment, and Challenge

During the time that AT&T underwent the largest corporate reorganization in history, Dr. Suzanne Kobasa studied the company's business executives. During this period of high stress and uncertainty, she observed that some executives stayed healthy while others experienced high levels of illness.

Kobasa discovered that the stress-resistant executives possessed a different kind of attitude about themselves and their life, which she termed "stress hardiness." She defined the stress-hardy personality as being characterized by three attitudes: control, commitment, and challenge. Specifically, stress-hardy individuals have a strong *commitment* to something outside of their self, a sense of *control* over events in their life, and an ability to view stress and change as *challenges* instead of threats. The "three Cs" prevent and minimize stress and its deleterious effects on well-being, sleep, and health.

Stress-hardy people are by nature optimistic. They see stressful situations as opportunities for growth and view change as normal and challenging. They are committed to something larger than themselves and take better advantage of social support.

In contrast, Kobasa found that the AT&T executives who became ill felt powerless, threatened, and debilitated by change and uncertainty. They retreated from stress and exhibited a sense of alienation from others.

What makes a person stress-hardy? Genetics, early life experiences, and parental influences all probably play a role. However, hardiness can also be learned using the following techniques, which promote the attitudes of control, commitment, and challenge:

1. Practice the relaxation response and cognitive restructuring. They will maximize a sense of control over your mind, body, stress, and life.
2. Instead of viewing change as a threat, view it as normal, constant, and a challenge. Change is stimulating, healthy, and essential for growth and personal development.
3. Be involved in something greater than yourself: work, family, community, religion. You will be less focused on yourself, which minimizes stress.

Develop a stress-hardy attitude. You will sleep better and your health and life will improve.

No Man Is an Island

Develop the attitude that "people need people," and you will reduce stress and its deleterious effects on sleep and health, boost the immune system, and probably live longer.

Substantial evidence indicates that people with adequate social support—defined as family, friends, community contacts, social or religious organizations, work relationships, or even a pet—are healthier, less likely to develop major and minor illnesses and mental health problems, and have a lower death rate. Specifically, studies show that social support provides this wide array of benefits:

- Reduced susceptibility to diseases of all types, from cancer to arthritis to heart disease
- Diminished risk of depression and stress-related illnesses
- Lessened risk of dying
- Lowered cholesterol

Once serious illness strikes, individuals with social support do better medically, recover more quickly, and have lower death rates. In a landmark study on women with breast cancer conducted at Stanford University, researchers found that those who participated in social support groups lived twice as long as those who did not. Social support may also be a key factor in reducing susceptibility to colds. In a 1997 study conducted by researchers at Carnegie-Mellon University, volunteers were intentionally dosed with a virus. The researchers found that the more diverse the subject's social relationships, the less likely he or she was to catch a cold.

Individuals who are socially isolated—who possess the belief that they have nobody with whom to share feelings or have close contact—are more likely to die earlier than those with strong social ties. This finding holds true regardless of race, ethnic background, sex, age, or socioeconomic status. People who live alone have more heart disease than those who live with someone or with a pet. In fact, inadequate social support is as dangerous to health as lack of exercise or high cholesterol and is as great or greater a risk factor for death than smoking!

Of course, isolation is not the same as solitude. Many people who live on their own are happy and healthy. It is the subjective sense of being isolated and alone, cut off from people and having no one to confide in, that is problematic. And not all social ties are health-enhancing. Some negative relationships, such as troubled or abusive ones, can be stress-inducing and associated with increased illness and suppression of immune functioning.

Nonetheless, there remains a significant advantage for those who have strong, stable connections to others. Furthermore, some studies show that just being married, whether satisfactorily or not, offers more protection from illness than no marriage at all.

A predisposition to social support is rooted in our biology: it was essential to our ancestors for hunting and gathering food, for protection from predators, and for survival. Social support begins with the attachment of child to parent. Studies consistently demonstrate that infants' mental and physical development are directly linked to adequate attachment and nurturing. Indeed, because we have the longest infancy in the animal kingdom, social attachment to our caregivers is a matter of life and death.

Social support provides many important health-enhancing benefits: affection, empathy, social activity, camaraderie, a sense of purpose and belonging. It also exerts positive effects on health because it allows us to:

- Share feelings and receive helpful suggestions
- Cope with stressful experiences
- Seek solutions to problems
- Reframe negative thoughts and change behavior
- Develop a sense of reliability and stability in times of transition
- Shift attention away from ourselves to something larger

Unfortunately, as science has discovered the importance of social relationships for health, society has caused an increase in social isolation and lack of connectedness. In the past several decades, social ties have been disrupted by mobility, fragmentation of the nuclear and extended family, single-parent families, and separations and divorces. Few have parents who live nearby or the same close-knit communities that existed in previous generations. Lifelong friendships are not as common. Most of us don't just drop over to a friend's house unannounced as was the case years ago.

If you don't have someone to go to when you are feeling upset, alone, or have a problem, here are ways to improve your social support network:

1. Practice all the techniques in this program for improving your sleep. As your sleep improves, so too will your mood. Consequently, you will attract supportive people more easily.

2. Join groups, clubs, or community organizations that interest you. Check the local newspaper, community events calendar, colleges, or religious organizations for information on these kinds of social groups.

3. If you are not allergic, get a pet. Pets can be a source of social support, affection, and good company. Studies show that pets lower the blood pressure of their owners and that pet owners have fewer doctor visits, lowered illness rates, higher survival rates for heart disease, and longer lives!
4. Avoid the tendency to withdraw under stress. Distract yourself and receive stress-reducing social support by seeking out family and friends and making an effort to socialize.
5. Instead of sitting home alone in your spare time watching television, call someone on the telephone, visit a neighbor, go to the health club, or go shopping or to dinner with someone.

Strong social ties can be powerful medicine. By building social ties and reducing feelings of isolation, you will improve your health and live longer. You will also reduce stress and minimize the likelihood that elevated stress hormones or feelings of loneliness will keep you awake at night.

Anger: The Unhealthy Emotion

Anger and other negative emotions are not always bad. Anger can be an appropriate response when being hurt, threatened, treated unjustly, demeaned, or blocked from realizing an important goal; it can right an injustice, mobilize others to change inappropriate behavior, and help us to accomplish goals.

For some, however, anger occurs too frequently and inappropriately. Excessive anger does not lead to positive behavioral change and becomes counterproductive and ineffective; it disturbs relationships, and only serves to heighten stress and impair mood.

When anger becomes chronic it can affect health, particularly when it takes the form of hostility—a more intense, pervasive, global type of anger that involves attitudes of cynicism, antagonism, or opposition. Angry people more easily elicit stress responses that cause blood pressure and heart rate to rise, blood cholesterol to increase, blood vessels to constrict, and oxygen flow to the heart to decrease. Angry people also take longer to recover from stress responses.

Consequently, of all the negative emotions, anger does the most harm to the heart and cardiovascular system. Research documents that people with high levels of anger and hostility are at greater risk for heart attacks and heart disease, and that reducing anger and hostility diminishes the risk of recurrent heart attack and may in fact prevent heart disease.

Chronic anger and hostility also weaken the immune system, adversely affect general health, and may even be life-threatening, as demonstrated by Dr. Redford Williams's finding at Duke University that hostile men are seven times more likely to die within twenty-five years (from any cause) than less hostile men. Angry people drive friends and family away and are more likely to reject the help of others, thereby reducing social support and placing the angry person's health in further jeopardy. Anger impairs the ability to think clearly, concentrate, and perform effectively. Because anger triggers the stress response, it disturbs sleep. Many of us have experienced nights when angry thoughts have kept us awake.

We are more prone to anger if stressed, irritated, or frustrated by something else. Thus, if someone is upset because the alarm didn't go off and is running late for an early meeting, there is more vulnerability to anger if the children are difficult during breakfast or a traffic jam occurs on the way to work.

Contrary to popular belief, men and women get angry equally often and as intensely. However, men are more likely to externalize their anger by yelling, throwing or slamming things, becoming aggressive, or drinking.

Fortunately, chronic anger is a habit that can be changed. We can learn to lower the threshold for anger and prevent and turn it off more easily. This takes considerable practice, but it can be done.

The first step in reducing anger is to take the attitude that anger is often maladaptive; the second is to practice the following techniques, which foster a less angry and hostile attitude in daily life:

1. Practice the relaxation response and cognitive restructuring, proven techniques for reducing anger. Regular practice of the relaxation response produces carry-over effects that reduce stress; consequently, our fuse isn't as short and our threshold for anger is higher. The relaxation response also quiets angry thoughts.

Cognitive restructuring reduces anger by reframing angry thoughts. Pay particular attention to the Cognitive Restructuring Diary described in the previous chapter; it can be used to spot patterns or situations that cause anger. By becoming more aware of these situations, you will be better able to control anger.

2. Practice the Stop-Mini-Reframe technique described in the previous chapter. It will help you develop a greater ability to turn off anger as it happens.

3. Don't expect perfection or that others will always meet your expectations. When perfectionism isn't achieved or the behavior of others does not live up to our expectations, anger results. Be realistic and modify expectations concerning perfectionism and the behavior of those around you.

4. In anger-producing situations, cool off by withdrawing, going off alone, using distraction, taking a walk or drive, or engaging in a pleasurable activity. Such activities quiet anger by preventing us from focusing on angry thoughts.

5. Exercise regularly. Exercise is an outlet for tension and produces a tranquilizing effect that reduces anger.

6. Practice empathy: see anger-producing interactions from the other person's perspective.

7. Develop a social support network. The support and caring of others can help reframe and short-circuit anger.

8. Follow basic religious and spiritual teachings: forgive when you feel you have been wronged and treat others as you would have them treat you. One reason religions stress these principles may be that they have known for centuries what science has only recently discovered—anger harms health and may be deadly.

9. Put anger in perspective by asking yourself how important an anger-producing situation would be if you had only one week to live. Many people who have had someone close to them die unexpectedly can put anger in perspective more easily.

With patience and regular practice of these techniques, anger can be reduced. Your mood, health, and relationships will improve, and you will be less likely to lie awake at night from elevated stress hormones or angry thoughts.

Laugh Your Stress Away

How often do you laugh? Recent studies document that taking a more humorous attitude toward ourselves and the world reduces stress and improves health.

Strong laughter numbs pain, produces a mild state of euphoria, and possibly also produces endorphins, the brain's opiatelike chemicals that produce a "high." Some studies have found that humor is as effective as the relaxation response in reducing stress and pain; others have found that humor boosts the functioning of the immune system.

The late Norman Cousins believed that he cured himself of a severe arthritic condition by using Marx Brothers and *Candid Camera* films to stimulate daily laughter. He found that ten minutes of hard laughter had an anesthetic effect that reduced pain and improved sleep.

Laughter reduces stress, anxiety, anger, and depression by allowing us to shift to a less serious perspective on ourselves and our lives. Seeing humor in a stressful situation provides a time-out from stress; it facilitates cognitive restructuring by reframing irrational thoughts and allowing a more positive way of viewing a situation.

Being able to use humor to laugh at ourselves is particularly stress-reducing, for it helps us to:

- Put our shortcomings into perspective and see that they are not so critical
- Lighten up and realize that none of us are perfect

- Take ourselves less seriously and be less concerned with ourselves

Laughter is also a great tension breaker and reduces barriers between people. By increasing a sense of connectedness, laughter reduces stress and increases positive emotions. Humor also increases a sense of empathy with others, which, as we have explored, is stress-reducing.

Children laugh freely and often. However, many of us lose touch with humor as we age. Some adults are so stressed and serious, they have forgotten how to laugh. Fortunately, using laughter and humor to reduce stress is a skill that can be learned. Here are some ways to develop a more humorous attitude in daily life:

- Read cartoons in newspapers, rent humorous videos, go to funny movies, or watch the comedy cable channel or late-night shows on television.
- Seek out funny people and avoid those who are too serious. When you hear a good joke, remember it and tell it to others.
- Get in touch with the child within and adopt an attitude of playfulness. Jump on a trampoline, swing on a swing set, play in the snow, engage in some silly games. Observe children and play with them; they are great teachers of humor.
- Research shows that by changing our facial expressions we can elicit corresponding emotions. Thus, by "putting on a smiling face," we can change our thoughts and make ourselves feel better. Conversely, a frown can make us feel sad. So pay attention to the facial expressions that you hold, for they affect how you feel. Every time you stand in front of a mirror, practice the habit of smiling so that it becomes more automatic.

Learn to laugh a lot. You will be more relaxed, healthier, and will sleep better. Being able you laugh at yourself will also increase self-esteem and confidence.

Help Yourself by Helping Others

Helping doesn't just feel good; studies show that it can reduce the effects of stress and improve the health of the helper. In one major study of 2,700 residents in Tecumseh, Michigan, researchers found that men who volunteered for community organizations were two and a half times less likely to die (from any cause) than men who did not volunteer. According to Drs. David Sobel and Robert Ornstein, authors of *The Healthy Mind, Healthy Body Handbook*, studies also show that helping is associated with boosted immune functioning, fewer colds and headaches, and relief from pain and insomnia.

The health-enhancing benefits of altruism may be the result of caring for someone else and seeing the benefits of our actions. Too much preoccupation with ourselves can lead to anxiety and depression by increasing concentration or problems; altruism reduces the focus on ourselves and serves as a distraction from problems and worries.

Altruism also reduces stress and its effects on sleep and health by providing the following benefits:

- Improved positive emotions such as caring
- Improved attitudes and feelings of greater contentment with what we have
- Increased self-esteem and sense of well-being by strengthening belief in our own skills and strengths
- Reduction in anger and social isolation and bolstering of social support

Allan Luks, author of *The Healing Power of Doing Good*, surveyed thousands of volunteers and discovered that practicing altruism on a regular basis provides an immediate, pleasurable sensation. This phenomenon, called helper's high, consists of sensations of warmth, increased energy, and euphoria, and can result in long-term effects of relaxation and calm.

Altruism is part of our biological evolution. Our ancestors survived by helping one another hunt, gather food, and defend against predators. Altruism is a way of feeling connected to something beyond ourselves, strengthening feelings of "we," and giving life meaning.

An altruistic attitude in daily life can be fostered by participating in many activities: tutoring, telephone work, visiting nursing homes, helping at hospitals or homeless shelters, cooking or delivering meals, or donating money. Some of these activities can be done alone; others may involve working with a community organization. The important thing is to choose an activity that you like and with which you feel comfortable.

Altruism can also be practiced by engaging in spontaneous acts of helping. Examples:

- Holding the door open for someone, assisting an elderly person, or helping someone whose arms are are full
- Letting another proceed ahead of you in line or in traffic
- Helping neighbors shovel their driveway after a snowstorm
- Sending a note or making a quick phone call to let someone know he or she did a good job

Develop an altruistic attitude in daily life. You will feel good, reduce stress, sleep better, and be healthier. You may also live longer.

Using Positive Illusions and Denial to Manage Stress

Psychologists have found that stress-resistant people are more than just optimistic: they distort reality and view it in the best possible light. Specifically, these individuals:

- Exaggerate how competent and well-liked they are
- Remember past behavior with a rosy glow

- Describe themselves primarily positively
- Exaggerate their belief in the control they have in what occurs around them

In short, stress-resistant individuals see themselves through positive illusions that are stress-reducing and mood- and health-enhancing. Because positive illusions are present in an even stronger degree in children, they may be evolutionary accommodations that are "wired in" and necessary for health.

To help themselves distort reality in a positive way, stress-resistant people minimize and negate stressful events by using denial. Traditionally, denial has been viewed as an unhealthy defense mechanism that prevents us from facing reality. Consequently, it has developed a negative reputation.

It is healthy and necessary to face up to major traumas, health problems, and other significant stressors. However, research on stress-resistant individuals indicates that denial of minor, everyday problems can he healthy. Minimizing, ignoring, or denying minor problems reduces stress and makes life more manageable. In contrast, being preoccupied with minor problems only serves to increase stress and its deleterious effects on mood, sleep, and health.

You can reduce stress, sleep better, and stay healthier if you use denial appropriately and shift beliefs about yourself toward positive illusions. Here are some strategies for promoting positive illusions:

1. Begin by recognizing and changing negative thinking. Practice the relaxation response and cognitive-restructuring techniques, which will help you minimize negative thinking and shift toward positive illusions.

2. Practice the techniques explored earlier in this chapter for developing optimism. Optimistic thinking promotes healthy positive illusions.

3. In daily life, many situations are ambiguous and can be perceived in many ways. Since we all distort reality through the mind's mental filters, choose the most positive perspective and distort reality in a positive way.

The Power and Biology of Faith

Throughout history, stress has been reduced by religious and spiritual beliefs. Recently science has begun to document that religious and spiritual beliefs may reduce stress and improve health. Consider the findings:

- Patients with religious beliefs are more likely to survive longer after cardiac surgery than those without religious beliefs.
- Religious and spiritual beliefs offer some protection from stress-related illnesses and cancer, and may lower death rates.
- Religious and spiritual beliefs are associated with reduced anxiety, anger, and depression, and with greater life and marital satisfaction, well-being, and self-esteem.
- The greater the elderly's religious involvement, the less their physical disability.
- People who attend religious services have lower blood pressure and half the risk of heart attack as nonattendees. In fact, religious beliefs may be as important in heart disease as traditional risk factors such as cholesterol and smoking!
- Religious beliefs are associated with fewer unhealthy behaviors such as smoking, drinking, and drug abuse.

The positive health effects of religious beliefs may be the result of the healthy habits that religions encourage, such as limiting smoking or alcohol intake. However, the effects may also be due to the fact that spiritual beliefs foster many of the stress-reducing attitudes and beliefs explored in this chapter: optimism; a sense of control, commitment, and challenge; empathy, forgiveness, and altruism.

Religious beliefs also reduce stress by providing a sense of meaning and purpose, placing stressors in perspective, and producing a calming effect that counters stress.

Dr. Herbert Benson of Harvard Medical School believes that religious beliefs and prayer may be health enhancing because they elicit the relaxation response. In fact, he believes that the tendency for humans to engage in religious beliefs and prayer may be encoded in our physiology for that evolutionary reason.

Consider finding and exploring suitable religious beliefs. By doing so, you will reduce stress and improve sleep and health.

The Week Six Progress Summary

The final progress summary, the Week Six Progress Summary, is included at the end of this chapter. It has one addition: an item for you to note improvements in daily life that result from practicing stress-resistant attitudes and beliefs. Examples:

- More optimistic, healthier thinking
- Enhanced control over stress and stress-related symptoms
- Reduced anger or heightened sense of humor
- Increased sense of connectedness to others
- More peace of mind

By reinforcing these improvements, you will boost confidence in your personal power and sleep better. You will also contribute to a healthier, more positive view of yourself and your life.

WEEK SIX PROGRESS SUMMARY

1. Assess your sleep pattern this week by noting:

a) the number of good nights of sleep ______________

b) the number of nights of core sleep (five and a half hours or more) ______________

c) the number of insomnia nights ______________

2. On how many daily sleep diaries did you record a positive sleep thought? ______________

3. How often did you mentally practice cognitive restructuring for negative sleep thoughts this week (circle one)?

regularly

occasionally

never

4. Assess your sleep-medication use this week by noting:

a) the number of medication-free nights ______________

b) the number of reduced-dosage nights ______________

c) the number of usual-dosage nights ______________

5. Track your sleep efficiency by calculating:

a) your average sleep time (number of hours per night) ______________

b) your average time in bed (number of hours per night) ______________

c) your average sleep efficiency (your average sleep time divided by your average time in bed) ______________

6. Track your sleep quality and the consistency of your rising time by noting:

a) your average sleep-quality rating from your sleep diaries ______________________

b) the number of days you arose within half an hour of your desired rising time ______________________

7. How often did you practice sleep-scheduling and stimulus-control techniques this week (circle one)?

regularly

occasionally

never

8. How often did you engage in sleep-enhancing lifestyle practices this week (circle one)?

regularly

occasionally

never

9. How often did you practice the relaxation response and minis during the day (circle one)?

regularly

occasionally

never

10. How often did you practice the relaxation response to help yourself fall asleep or back to sleep at night (circle one)?

regularly

occasionally

never

11. How often did you practice cognitive restructuring for stress management this week (circle one)?

regularly

occasionally

never

12. How often did you practice stress-reducing attitudes and beliefs this week (circle one)?

regularly

occasionally

never

13. Check all areas of progress listed below that you have made since beginning this program:

______ experiencing fewer insomnia nights

______ experiencing more nights of core sleep

______ experiencing more nights of good sleep

______ falling asleep faster

______ waking less often during the night

______ waking for shorter periods of time during the night

______ averaging more sleep time per night

______ improved quality of sleep

______ improved sleep efficiency

______ decreased sleep medication

14. Summarize any positive changes you noticed in yourself and your life as a result of this program:

____

____

____

____

Appendix A: Managing Shift Work

Millions of people work the night, or "graveyard," shift (11:00 P.M. to 7:00 A.M.) or rotate among day, evening, and night shifts. More than half of these workers experience sleep difficulties. Studies demonstrate that shift workers experience poorer sleep quality, shorter sleep, and more difficulty falling asleep and staying asleep than regular day workers.

Why is short work associated with such a high incidence of sleep problems? Recall from chapter 2 that body temperature, which plays an important role in promoting sleep and wakefulness, is directly influenced by the daily cycles of light and darkness. Light causes body temperature to rise (which promotes wakefulness), while darkness causes temperature to fall (which promotes sleep). Thus, night and rotating shift workers are more prone to sleep disturbances because they must usually sleep during the day—the time when nature intended us to be awake.

Shift workers must also work when our bodies were designed to be asleep. Consequently, they are more likely to be drowsy or fall asleep during work. Studies have shown that 75 percent of night workers feel drowsy at work and that over half admit to falling asleep on the job. (In fact, it is not uncommon for night workers to doze off while driving home from work.)

Reduced alertness on the job impairs performance, productivity, and work quality and increases chances of error, safety problems, and on-the-job accidents. In fact, a number of serious industrial accidents have been related to fatigue and sleepiness during the night shift. The near meltdown that occurred in 1979 at the Three Mile Island nuclear power plant occurred at 4:00 A.M. and involved a work crew that had just changed to the graveyard shift. Other accidents attributed to shift work include the *Exxon Valdez* oil spill and the Chernobyl nuclear disaster.

Shift workers report higher levels of job dissatisfaction, absenteeism, and low morale. Shift work is associated with increased use of sleeping pills and alcohol to aid sleep as well as stimulants such as caffeine to stay awake. Mood and general health and well-being are poorer and levels of stress are higher among night and rotating shift workers compared to day workers.

Because someone on the graveyard shift has less time to spend with a spouse and children, marital and family relationships suffer. When shift workers try to socialize with family and friends on days off, they often lack the energy and enthusiasm to enjoy social interaction. And since there is less time to socialize in general, social isolation and loneliness become problematic.

Working the night shift is difficult enough, but rotating among day, night, and evening shifts is worse; it is like working for a week in the United States, a week in Europe, then a week in Asia—a type of jet lag without flying. When the body must quickly adjust to a new waking and sleeping schedule, it never has a chance to adjust to one shift and establish a consistent body-temperature rhythm.

When rotating shifts are repeated month after month, the resulting chronic disruption in the body-temperature rhythm almost guarantees disturbed sleep and reduced alertness. Consequently, those on rotating shifts encounter even greater disruptions in sleep, alertness, and mood than regular night shift workers.

Some people adjust more easily to shift work than others; it is hardest on insomniacs, who have a sensitive sleep system to begin with, and older people, whose body-temperature rhythms have a harder time adjusting than those of younger people.

If you work the night shift, the following guidelines will minimize its deleterious effects:

1. Try to maintain the same sleep-wake schedule on your days off. This will give your body regular cues (such as a consistent rising time and regular periods of physical and social activity) that will synchronize your body-temperature rhythm. Unfortunately, this practice is difficult for most shift workers since they socialize on a conventional schedule on their days off.

2. When leaving work in the morning, wear dark glasses to prevent sunlight from causing your body temperature and alertness level to increase.

3. Allow sufficient time to wind down after work. If you get off work at 7:00 A.M., do not attempt to go to sleep at 8:00 A.M.

4. Ensure that your sleep will not be interrupted by light, doorbells, telephones, noises from the street, or people. Darken your bedroom by using dark drapes or an eyeshade. Don't let children, your spouse, or the telephone interrupt your sleep. Use a sound conditioner, fan, or earplugs to reduce noise and place rugs on wooden floors to deaden the sound of footsteps. Review chapter 7 concerning other guidelines for creating an optimal sleep environment.

5. Practice the techniques in this program for improving sleep; they will minimize the sleep disruptions caused by night work.

6. Get together with your coworkers and suggest to your employer that your work environment be equipped with bright light. Bright light increases alertness and performance on the job (which may increase your employer's profits and compensate for the cost of the lights); it also synchronizes the body-temperature rhythm so that you will sleep better during the day.

The deleterious effects of rotating shifts can be minimized by preparing for a shift change in advance; that is, by adjusting bedtimes and wake-up times a few days prior to the new shift. For example, a few days before switching from the evening shift (3:00 P.M. to 11:00 P.M.) to the night shift (11:00 P.M. to 7:00 A.M.), set bedtimes and wake-up times a few hours later; when changing from the night to day shift, move bedtimes and wake-up times a few hours earlier. Expose yourself to bright light when you rise from bed and during work to promote wakefulness.

Rotating shift workers should also avoid exposure to bright light during the few hours before bedtime so that the body doesn't think it is time to wake up. Sleep disruptions from rotating shifts can also be minimized by paying particular attention to creating an ideal sleep environment and practicing all the techniques in this program for improving sleep.

Appendix B: Managing Jet Lag

Jet lag, a consequence of travel by jet aircraft, is a combination of symptoms that are experienced when flying across several time zones. The symptoms of jet lag include:

- Sleepiness during the day
- Difficulty falling or staying asleep at night
- Gastrointestinal disturbances such as upset stomach, diarrhea, or constipation
- Fatigue, malaise, and achiness
- Disorientation, confusion, difficulty concentrating, irritability, distorted sense of time, and slowed mental reactions

To understand why jet lag occurs, let's suppose you fly from Boston at 9:00 P.M. and arrive in London at 9:00 A.M. local time. Because your are still on Boston time, your body temperature would think it is 3:00 A.M. Consequently, you would feel sleepy, lethargic, disoriented, and would not think clearly—not the best conditions for driving in London rush-hour traffic or enjoying the first day of a vacation. If you tried to go to sleep at 11:00 P.M.

London time, your body would think it was 3:00 P.M. and you would have a difficult time falling asleep.

When flying west, the opposite problem occurs. Flying from Boston to Los Angeles, my body would think it is 11:00 P.M. when it is 8:00 P.M. Los Angeles time; consequently, I would have a difficult time staying awake and would probably awaken in the early morning hours. Insomnia is usually more problematic with eastbound flights because our body clock lags behind local time, meaning that we must force sleep if we are to conform to the local schedule.

The duration and severity of jet lag symptoms increase with the number of time zones crossed. While crossing one or two time zones does not usually create much of a problem with jet lag, crossing three time zones does, although the symptoms persist for only a few days. In contrast, flying halfway around the world can produce symptoms that last for weeks. Being unable to sleep comfortably on airplanes, coupled with the stress of traveling, exacerbates jet lag symptoms.

In general, we require about one day per time zone crossed to synchronize our body-temperature rhythm to the new time zone. Thus, someone who travels from America to Asia for a one-week stay may have jet lag for the entire visit.

If you are a business traveler flying across several time zones but plan to stay at your destination for only a day or two, the trip won't be long enough to permit you to adjust to the new time. Therefore, you are better off maintaining your normal sleep-wake schedule as much as possible and trying to conduct business while you are awake and alert. (That's why pilots usually try to maintain their home sleep schedule when they are on quick-turnaround flights.) It is important to ensure that your sleeping quarters are shielded from light and sound as much as possible during local daytime hours.

Business travelers or vacationers who cross several time zones and plan to spend more than a few days at their destination will experience more problems with jet lag. Therefore, they should try to adjust to the new time as quickly as possible. The following steps can be taken before, during, and after a flight to hasten this adjustment and minimize jet lag:

1. Before leaving, gradually adjust your bedtimes, rising times, and mealtimes to the time zone of your destination. For eastbound flights, this means rising, eating, and going to bed earlier; for westbound flights, go to bed, eat, and rise later. The further in advance your adjust these times, the more you will minimize jet lag.
2. During the flight, drink plenty of fluids to prevent dehydration due to the plane's low humidity (pressurized air in airplanes is very dry). Dehydration makes it more difficult for body temperature to adjust to the new time zone. Avoid alcohol and caffeine on the flight; these substances exacerbate dehydration.
3. A sleeping pill may make it easier to sleep on the plane and adjust to the new time zone. A short-acting sleeping pill (see chapter 3) is best because it will work and be eliminated quickly from your body.
4. Upon arrival in the new time zone, immediately adjust your sleep schedule to the local time. For example, if arriving in London at 9:00 A.M., don't sleep during the day, even though your body says its 3:00 A.M. Boston time. Stay outside and use exposure to sunlight, physical activity, and social contact to prevent drowsiness. If you are indoors, stay near windows or in rooms with lots of sunlight. Schedule meals at the proper local time.
5. Try not to go to bed until it is appropriate for the local time zone. If necessary, take a short nap to help you get through the day. Make sure your room is dark to minimize nighttime awakenings.
6. Give yourself time to adjust to the new time zone and don't schedule much the first day. If you are on business, arrive a day or two before meetings if possible. For the first day or two, schedule meetings when you would be awake at home.
7. If you are a business traveler who regularly crosses many time zones, consider purchasing a light box. As previously discussed, light boxes are relatively inexpensive and can be used to delay or advance body-temperature changes. Some studies with air travelers and pilots document

that exposure to bright-light boxes several days before departure (morning exposure for eastbound flights, evening exposure for westbound flights) can speed up synchronization with the local time and reduce jet lag. (Several companies have even developed a baseball-type cap outfitted with bright lights that can be used while flying and upon arrival to shift body temperature to match local time.)

Whether you are a vacationer or business traveler crossing several time zones, these guidelines will minimize jet lag and make your trip more enjoyable and productive.

Appendix C: Infants' and Children's Sleep

Some children seem to be born good sleepers; they fall asleep easily and sleep soundly throughout the night. Others have difficulty sleeping from the time they are born, experiencing problems falling asleep, staying asleep, or both. These sleep problems can be quite stressful for parents. In fact, some insomniacs trace the beginning of their sleep problems to the disrupted nights caused by their child's sleep difficulties.

Compared to adult studies, there has been far less research on children's sleep problems. Fortunately, there has been a significant increase in research on infant, child, and adolescent sleep in the past few years. We now know that although children may inherit a tendency toward being good or poor sleepers, learning factors also play an important role and that children can learn to be better sleepers.

Infants

Although newborns sleep on and off throughout a twenty-four-hour day, they begin to develop a more consistent sleep-wake rhythm a few months after birth that corresponds to day and night. Although most infants begin to sleep through the night at this time, many have difficulty falling asleep on their own at bedtime; others continue to have difficulty sleeping through the night or can't fall back to sleep by themselves.

You can help your infant to fall asleep on his or her own and sleep more soundly during the night by following these guidelines:

1. Expose infants to bright light, activity, and stimulation during the day and darkness and quiet at night; this helps infants to learn the difference between day and night and to establish a consistent body-temperature rhythm. As infants get older, shorten the length of their naps by waking them; this will increase the pressure for sleep at night and help infants to learn that nighttime is for sleeping.

2. Just as many adults need a quiet wind-down period before bedtime, so do infants. This period should be enjoyable, predictable, and consistent by a few months of age. Turning down the lights and engaging in quiet activities such as reading books, singing lullabies, or just quiet talking are all effective wind-down activities.

3. Make sure the infant's room is sufficiently quiet and dark at night. When she or he needs to be fed or changed during the night, limit noise, movement, talking, and other stimulation. Gradually reduce the frequency of nighttime feedings and lengthen the time between them, which will minimize awakenings. Most babies no longer require nighttime feedings after six months.

4. One of the most important things a baby can learn is to fall asleep on his or her own. Therefore, infants should be put in the crib before they fall asleep so that they learn to associate the crib with falling asleep. Similarly, a child who awakens during the night should learn to fall back to sleep in the crib. Be careful about letting a nursing baby fall asleep on the mother's chest; with such a warm and comfortable place to sleep, it is easy to understand why the baby will learn not to sleep in the crib.

Obviously, an infant who cries at bedtime or during the night needs to be comforted. However, at about three to six months of age, the infant should be taught to fall asleep on his or her own instead of depending upon a bottle, being held, or sleeping in your bed.

Dr. Richard Ferber, a pediatrician at Harvard Medical School's Children's Hospital and author of *Solve Your Child's Sleep Problems*, has helped many parents (my wife and me included!) teach their infants good sleeping habits. Ferber recommends this progressive schedule for teaching infants ages three to six months to fall asleep on their own:

1. If a baby cries at bedtime or after a nighttime awakening, let the child cry for five minutes. Then go into the baby's room, reassure the baby by talking softly, and leave the room. Don't reinforce the baby's crying by picking the baby up, massaging or patting the baby, or spending more than a few minutes in the room.
2. If the baby continues to cry, let the crying continue for ten minutes, then return to the room. Reassure the baby without picking him or her up, then leave the room quickly. If the baby continues to cry, return to the bedroom after fifteen minutes of crying. Subsequent checks should be after an additional fifteen minutes of crying.
3. The following night, the first check should be after ten minutes of crying; the second check after fifteen minutes; and subsequent checks after twenty minutes. For each successive night, add five minutes to the length of the first and subsequent checks.

With this method, most babies learn to fall asleep on their own within a week (it sometimes takes the parents that long to get comfortable with the idea of letting the baby cry for more than a few minutes). In some instances, the baby may cry for as much as an hour or two the first or second night; however, the duration of crying usually diminishes on each successive night. The key to succeeding with Ferber's approach is consistency and a willingness to lose some sleep the first few nights of implementing it (that's why many parents find that weekend nights are good nights to start Ferber's method).

As infants get older, it is a good idea to let them sleep with a stuffed animal or soft "attachment object" such as a blanket. Over time, the infant will learn to associate falling asleep with the animal or object rather than with you.

Preschool and School-Age Children

Somewhere between 20 and 25 percent of preschool and school-age children have sleep problems such as difficulty going to bed and falling or staying asleep, needing a lot of attention to fall asleep at bedtime, or needing to sleep in another room or in their parents' bed. Often these children did not learn good sleep habits as infants.

The following guidelines for preschoolers and school-age children will ensure good sleep patterns:

1. Although children exhibit wide differences in how frequently and long they nap, most outgrow naps between three and six years of age. Until then, naps should be taken in the early afternoon and limited to two hours. Otherwise, your child may not feel drowsy at the usual bedtime.

2. Since physical activity promotes sound sleep, make sure your child gets plenty of exercise. Health officials are concerned about the fact that an increasing percentage of children are sedentary. The primary culprit is television; it is not uncommon for some children to watch three or more hours of television each day. Limiting children's television time and encouraging physical activity, especially in the late afternoon or early evening, will improve their sleep.

3. Limit your child's consumption of caffeinated foods and beverages. Caffeine has a far greater stimulant effect on children than on adults and therefore disturbs children's sleep more easily. Colas, chocolates (candy, ice cream, cocoa), and other caffeine-containing substances should be avoided after lunchtime.

4. Give your child a relaxing wind-down period before bedtime. Limit noise, excitement, and physical activity during this time and encourage your child to engage in quiet, relaxing activities such a reading or quiet play.

5. Establish a regular and predictable bedtime routine that will help your child associate bedtime with sleep. This routine might include brushing teeth, reading a book, preparing the bed with a favorite stuffed animal, turning down the lights, and a goodnight hug or kiss. Be sure to allow sufficient time (usually twenty to thirty minutes) for this routine.

6. Set a regular bedtime that corresponds with the time your child normally feels sleepy. However, if your child is not sleepy at bedtime, allow an extra fifteen minutes to read a book. Otherwise, the child may begin to associate bedtime with a frustrating inability to fall asleep.

Also, be careful about promoting negative sleep thoughts such as "if you don't get a good night's sleep, you will feel exhausted tomorrow." Otherwise, your child may begin to feel anxious and pressured about sleep, which will only increase the likelihood of chronic sleep problems. In most cases, you can rest assured that your child will get the amount of sleep he or she requires and will sleep when necessary.

7. If your child can't fall asleep at a reasonable time, gradually establish an earlier morning wake-up time. This will advance the child's body-temperature rhythm so that he or she will fall asleep earlier at night. Also, maintain a consistent rising time; this will help your child to feel sleepy at a regular time each night.

8. Once your child is in bed, avoid letting him or her get out of bed for "one more drink of water" or "one more hug." The more consistently you reinforce these behaviors, the more your child will learn to test the limits by getting out of bed. Put your child back in bed quickly and without much discussion. Use verbal reward and consider using a reward in the morning such as a treat or activity if your child exhibits positive bedtime behaviors.

9. Don't put children to bed early as a punishment. If a child goes to bed upset, he or she will have difficulty falling asleep and will feel negative about bedtime. Your child should associate the bed and bedtime with sleep, not punishment.

Finally, your child may go through periods when he or she is afraid to go to bed because of fears of the dark, monsters, or nightmares. It is important that you don't allow your child to escape fears by sleeping in your bed or another room; this will reinforce your child's belief that he or she can't sleep alone.

Here are several strategies for teaching your child to deal with nighttime fears:

- Allow your child to leave a night-light on or the door partially open, then gradually reduce the amount of light or the degree that the door is open
- Teach your child relaxation and pleasant imagery techniques (favorite place or fantasy hero) to use at bedtime; these techniques will relax and distract your child from anxious thoughts
- Limit your child's exposure to frightening images on television or videotapes
- Explain the differences between fantasy and reality to your child

Teaching children to sleep well involves time and patience but is well worth the effort, as they will learn good sleep habits that will ensure sound sleep for the rest of their lives.

Appendix D: Additional Relaxation Scripts

Autogenic Training

Autogenic training is a relaxation technique that was developed in Germany by Dr. Johannes Schultz. Autogenic means "self-induced"; it self-induces relaxation by utilizing suggestions of warmth and heaviness. The following script is a modified version of Dr. Schultz's original autogenic training.

> Close your eyes and direct your attention to the toes and feet. Feel a wave of relaxation begin to move through the feet. Now the relaxation moves through the calves and thighs, then to the stomach, chest, and back. Note tension disappearing from your body. Sense relaxation moving now to the hands, forearms, upper arms, and shoulders. Next the relaxation moves to the neck, jaw, cheeks, eyes, and forehead. Tension is disappearing from the body.
>
> Focus your attention on your breathing. Note that the breathing is becoming more rhythmic and abdominal.

As you inhale, the stomach expands; as you exhale, it contracts. Take a few moments to concentrate on abdominal breathing.

If your mind wanders to distracting thoughts, gently let the thoughts go and return your attention to the breathing. It may help to repeat a word silently to yourself each time that you exhale, such as *one* or *relax*. This word will serve as a mental focus to direct the mind away from distracting, everyday thoughts. Take a few moments to concentrate on breathing and the word.

Now that your breathing has become more rhythmic and abdominal, direct your attention to the arms. As you focus on the arms, repeat slowly to yourself "My arms are heavy." It may help to visualize an image of the arms becoming heavy. Slowly repeat "My arms are heavy" two more times. Direct your attention now to the legs and slowly repeat to yourself "My legs are heavy." Again, it may help to visualize the legs becoming heavy. Slowly repeat "My legs are heavy" two more times.

Concentrate your attention now back to your arms and repeat slowly to yourself "My arms are warm." Visualize an image of the arms becoming warm. Slowly repeat "My arms are warm" two more times. Focus next on the legs and repeat slowly to yourself "My legs are warm," visualizing the legs becoming warm. Slowly repeat "My legs are warm" two more times.

Your entire body is heavier, warmer, and more relaxed. Take a few moments to note the absence of tension throughout the body. You feel calm, relaxed, and peaceful.

Finally, at your own pace, take a slow, deep breath and slowly open your eyes.

Nature Scene

The following relaxation script incorporates visualization of a relaxing place in nature to elicit the relaxation response.

> Close your eyes and direct your attention to the toes and feet. Feel a wave of relaxation begin to move through the feet. Now the relaxation moves through the calves and thighs, then to the stomach, chest, and back. Note tension disappearing from your body. Sense relaxation moving now to the hands, forearms, upper arms, and shoulders. Next the relaxation moves to the neck, jaw, cheeks, eyes, and forehead. Tension is disappearing from the body.
>
> Concentrate now on the breathing. Note that the breathing is becoming more rhythmic and abdominal. Also notice that, as your inhale, the stomach expands; as you exhale, it contracts. Take a few moments to focus on abdominal breathing.
>
> If the mind drifts to distracting thoughts, let the thoughts go and return your attention to breathing. It may help to repeat a word silently to yourself each time that you exhale, such as *one* or *relax*. This word will serve as a mental focus to direct the mind away from distracting thoughts. Take a few moments to concentrate on breathing and the word.
>
> Now that you are relaxing more deeply, imagine yourself in a tranquil place in nature, one that you have visited or would like to visit: a meadow, a beach, a mountain. Take a few moments to consider the beauty: the sky, trees, animals, flowers, or whatever you observe. Are there any sounds such as water, wind, or birds, or any smells such as flowers or grass? Sense the warmth of the sun against your skin. Take a few moments to be at peace in this soothing environment.

Now sit or lie down in this serene place. Look up and notice the sky, clouds, or perhaps the moon or stars. You are becoming more deeply relaxed. You feel calm and peaceful. Take a few moments to enjoy this safe and wonderful place, which you can return to anytime that you need to relax.

Take one more look around, then take a slow, deep breath and slowly open your eyes.

Progressive Relaxation

Progressive relaxation is a technique that was developed by Dr. Edmund Jacobsen and described in his book *Progressive Relaxation.* This technique involves tensing and relaxing the muscles throughout the body to increase awareness of tension and relaxation and to elicit the relaxation response. The following script is a modified version of Dr. Jacobsen's original technique.

Close your eyes and direct your attention to your breathing. Allow the breathing to become slower and more rhythmic. Notice the abdomen expand as you inhale and contract as you exhale. Take a few moments to concentrate on breathing.

Now that you are relaxing, clench the right fist. Clench tighter and tighter, noting the tension in the right hand. Hold the tension for about five seconds, then quickly release the tension and allow the right hand to relax. Note the sense of relaxation in the right hand and how this differs from tension. Repeat the tense-relax procedure with the left hand.

Next tense your right arm. Hold the tension for above five seconds and note that feeling of tension. Now release the tension quickly and focus on the sense of relaxation in the right arm. Be aware of how this sensation differs from tension. Repeat the tense-relax procedure with the left arm.

Focus now on your right leg. Tense the leg, hold the tension, then release it quickly. Concentrate on the feeling of relaxation in the right leg and how this differs from tension. Repeat the tense-relax procedure with the left leg.

The muscles are becoming more relaxed and the breathing slower and more rhythmic. If your mind drifts to distracting thoughts, return your attention to the feeling of relaxation in the body.

Now tense the abdomen. Hold the tension for five seconds and notice the feeling of tension in the abdomen. Quickly release the tension and be aware of how relaxation differs from tension. Repeat the tense-relax procedure for the back muscles, noting the difference between tension and relaxation. Tense and relax the neck and shoulder muscles, then the jaw, cheeks, eyes, and forehead, concentrating on the difference between tension and relaxation in these muscles.

Spend a few moments feeling relaxation in your body. Note the slower rhythmic breathing pattern. Disregard any distracting thoughts. You are becoming more deeply relaxed, calm, and peaceful. Take a few moments to concentrate on relaxation.

Finally, at your own pace, take a slow, deep breath and slowly open your eyes.

Sources and Suggested Reading

Introduction

Benson, H., M. Malholtra, R. Goldman, G. Jacobs, and P. Hopkins (1990). Three case reports of the metabolic and electroencephalographic changes associated with advanced buddhist meditation techniques. *Behavioral Medicine,* 16: 90–95.

Jacobs, G. D., R. Heilbronner, and J. Stanley (1984). The effects of short-term flotation REST on relaxation: a controlled study. *Health Psychology,* 3(2): 99–112.

Jacobs G. D., and J. F. Lubar (1989). Spectral analyses of the central nervous system effects of the relaxation response elicited by autogenic training. *Behavioral Medicine,* 15: 125–132.

Wake Up America: A National Sleep Alert (January 1993). Report of the National Commission on Sleep Disorders Research submitted to the United States Congress and to the Secretary, U.S. Department of Health and Human Services.

Chapter 1

Everitt, D.E., and Avorn, J. (1990). Clinical decision making in the treatment of insomnia. *The American Journal of Medicine,* 89: 357–362.

Jacobs, G. D., H. Benson, and R. Friedman (1996). Perceived benefits in a behavioral medicine insomnia program: a clinical report. *American Journal of Medicine,* 100: 212–216.

Jacobs, G. D., R. Friedman, and H. Benson (1993). Home-based central nervous system assessment of a multifactor behavioral intervention for chronic sleep-onset insomnia. *Behavior Therapy,* 24: 159–174.

Jacobs, G. D., P. Rosenberg, R. Friedman, et al. (1993). Multifactor behavioral treatment of chronic sleep-onset insomnia using stimulus control and the relaxation response. *Behavior Modification,* 17: 498–509.

Morin, Charles (1993). *Insomnia: Psychological Assessment and Management.* New York: Guilford Press.

Morin, C. M., J. P. Culbert, and S. M. Schwartz (1994). Nonpharmacological interventions for insomnia: a meta-analysis of treatment efficacy. *American Journal of Psychiatry,* 151(8): 1172–1180.

Morin, C. M., and J. A. Kwentus (1988). Behavioral and pharmacological treatments for insomnia. *Annals of Behavioral Medicine,* 10(3): 91–97.

Schorr, R. I., and S. F. Bauwens (1992). Diagnosis and treatment of outpatient insomnia by psychiatric and nonpsychiatric physicians. *The American Journal of Medicine,* 93: 78–82.

Chapter 2

Dotto, L. (1990). *Losing Sleep: How Your Sleeping Habits Affect Your Life.* New York: William Morrow.

Morin, C. M. (1993). *Insomnia: Psychological Assessment and Management.* New York: Guilford Press.

Morris, M., L. Lack, and D. Dawson (1990). Sleep-onset insomniacs have delayed temperature rhythms. *Sleep,* 13(1): 1–14.

Prinz, P. N., M. V. Vitiello, M. A. Raskind, and M. J. Thorpy (1990). Geriatrics: sleep disorders and aging. *The New England Journal of Medicine,* 323(8): 520–525.

Sewitch, D. (1987). Slow wave sleep deficiency insomnia: a problem in thermo-downregulation at sleep onset. *Psychophysiology,* 24: 200–215.

Soldatos, C. (1994). Insomnia in relation to depression and anxiety: epidemiologic considerations. *Journal of Psychosomatic Research,* 38(1): 3–8.

Chapter 3

Brezinski, A. (1997). Melatonin in humans. *New England Journal of Medicine,* 336(3): 186–195.

Gillin, J. C. (1991). The long and short of sleeping pills. *New England Journal of Medicine,* 324(24): 1735–1736.

Wysowski, D. K., and C. Baum (1991). Outpatient use of prescription sedative-hypnotic drugs in the United States, 1970 through 1989. *Archives of Internal Medicine,* 151: 1779–1784.

Chapter 4

Barlow, D.H., and M. Craske (1994). *Mastery of Your Anxiety and Panic.* Albany, New York: Graywind Publications.

Beck, A. (1976). *Cognitive Therapy and the Emotional Disorders.* New York: International Universities Press.

Copeland, M. A. (1992). *The Depression Workbook.* Oakland, CA: New Harbinger.

Gillin, J. C., and W. F. Byerley (1990). The diagnosis and management of insomnia. *New England Journal of Medicine,* 322(4): 239–248.

Kupfer, D., and C. F. Reynolds (1997). Management of insomnia. *The New England Journal of Medicine,* 336: 341–346.

Meichenbaum, D. (1977). *Cognitive Behavior Modification: An Integrative Approach.* New York: Plenum Press.

Chapter 5

Benson, H., and M. Epstein (1975). The placebo effect: a neglected asset in the care of patients. *Journal of the American Medical Association,* 232: 1225–1227.

Kiecolt-Glaser, J. K., and R. Glaser (1988). Psychological influences on immunity. *American Psychologist,* 43: 892–898.

Stampi, C. (1989). Ultrashort sleep/wake patterns and sustained performance. In *Sleep and Alertness: Chronobiological, Behavioral, and Medical Aspects of Napping.* Edited by D. Dinges and R. Broughton. New York: Raven Press.

Stepanski, E. et. al. (1988). Daytime alertness in patients with chronic insomnia compared to asymptomatic control subjects. *Sleep,* 11(1): 54–60.

Webb, W. B., and H. W. Agnew (1974). The effects of chronic limitation of sleep length. *Psychophysiology,* 11(3): 265–272.

Chapter 6

Bootzin, R. R., M. Engle-Friedman, and L. Hazelwood (1983). Insomnia. In *Clinical Geropsychology: New Directions in Assessment and Treatment.* Edited by P. M. Lewinsohn and L. Teri. New York: Pergamon Press.

Campbell, S. S., and J. Zulley (1985). Ultradian components of human sleep/wake patterns during disentrainment. *Experimental Brain Research* supplement, 12: 234–255.

Dinges, D., and R. Broughton, eds. (1989). *Sleep and Alertness: Chronobiological, Behavioral, and Medical Aspects of Napping.* New York: Raven Press.

Spielman, A. J., P. Saskin, and M. J. Thorpy (1987). Treatment of insomnia by restriction of time in bed. *Sleep,* 10(1): 45–56.

Chapter 7

Ferguson, T. (1987). *The No-Nag, No-Guilt, Do-It-Your-Own Way Guide to Quitting Smoking.* New York: Ballantine.

King, A. C. et al. (1997). Moderate intensity exercise and self-rated quality of sleep in older adults. *Journal of the American Medical Association,* 277(1): 32–37.

Pate, R. R. et al. (1995). Physical activity and public health. *Journal of the American Medical Association,* 273(5): 402–407.

Rippe, J. M., and A. Ward (1989). *Dr. James Rippe's Complete Book of Fitness Walking.* New York: Prentice Hall.

Rosenthal, N. (1993). *Winter Blues: What It Is and How to Overcome It.* New York: Guilford Press.

Chapter 8

Benson, H. (1975). *The Relaxation Response.* New York: William Morrow.

Benson, H., and E. Stuart (1992). *The Wellness Book.* New York: Fireside.

Borysenko, J. (1987). *Minding the Body, Mending the Mind.* Reading, MA: Addison Wesley.

Goleman, D., and J. Gurin (1993). *Mind Body Medicine: How to Use Your Mind for Better Health.* New York: Consumer Reports Books.

Pelletier, K. (1977). *Mind As Healer, Mind As Slayer.* New York: Dell Publishing.

Selye, H. (1956). *The Stress of Life.* New York: McGraw-Hill.

Chapter 9

Burns, D. (1989). *The Feeling Good Handbook.* New York: Plume.

Ellis, A., and R. Greiger (1977). *Handbook of Rationale Emotive Therapy.* New York: Springer.

LeDoux, Joseph (1996). *The Emotional Brain.* New York: Simon & Schuster.

Meichenbaum, D. (1985). *Stress Inoculation Training.* New York: Pergamon Press.

Chapter 10

Baim, M., and L. La Roche (1992). Jest 'n' Joy. In H. Benson and E. Stuart, *The Wellness Book*. New York: Fireside.

Benson, H. (1996). *Timeless Healing: The Power and Biology of Belief.* New York: Scribner.

Luks, A. (1991). *The Healing Power of Doing Good: The Health and Spiritual Benefits of Helping Others.* New York: Fawcett Columbine.

Maddi, S., and S. Kobasa (1984). *The Hardy Executive: Health Under Stress.* Chicago: Dorsey Professional Books.

Seligman, M. (1990). *Learned Optimism.* New York: Knopf.

Sobel, D., and R. Ornstein (1996). *The Healthy Mind, Healthy Body Handbook.* Los Altos, CA: DRx.

Williams, R. (1989). *The Trusting Heart.* New York: Times Books.

How to Order Dr. Jacobs's Relaxation Response Tape

Dr. Jacobs's twenty-minute relaxation response tape is $10.00 (including shipping and handling). To order a tape, please mail a check (or money order if you live outside the United States) made payable to Dr. Gregg Jacobs to:

Dr. Gregg Jacobs
110 Francis Street, Suite 1A
Boston, MA 02215
(617) 632-7369

Please include your name and address and allow two to three weeks for delivery.

Acknowledgments

As an undergraduate at Lawrence University in Appleton, Wisconsin, I was fortunate to have two professors, Dr. John Stanley and Dr. Bruce Hetzler, who through their courses introduced me to the emerging field of behavioral medicine. They encouraged my interest in the field, sponsored my tutorials, independent studies, and honors thesis, and worked closely and patiently with me during my years at Lawrence. Their influence on my thinking and my career was tremendous and I will always be grateful to them.

I am also grateful to Dr. Richard Warch, President of Lawrence University, who supported my research there. My years at Lawrence stimulated my thinking, provided me with the skills to become a clinician and scientist, and were nothing less than enchanting.

Dr. Allan Belden and John Kemp gave me my first opportunity to work with patients by hiring me as a stress management specialist at St. Elizabeth's Hospital in Appleton. Their support, guidance, and confidence in me were greatly appreciated. I also thank Dr. Joel Lubar for the opportunity to work with him and complete my doctoral degree at the University of Tennessee. His instruction and wisdom prepared me for a career as a scientist and clinician.

I am indebted to the pioneering work of several individuals, including Dr. Herbert Benson, Dr. Kenneth Pelletier, Dr. Robert Ornstein, and Dr. David Sobel, who influenced my thinking early in my career and have contributed enormously to the field of behavioral and mind-body medicine. Herbert Benson also gave me the opportunity to work with him as a postdoctoral fellow at Harvard Medical School and to continue my work with him for the past eleven years. He provided me with the initial support needed to continue my research and has been a mentor, colleague, and friend. It has been an inspiration and privilege to work with him.

Dr. Dennis Russo and Dr. Bruce Masek provided me with the opportunity to receive clinical training at Harvard Medical School's Children's Hospital as a postdoctoral fellow. Their encouragement, guidance, and knowledge as clinicians helped shape my career and the career of many others.

I am also grateful to my colleagues at the Division of Behavioral Medicine, the Mind/Body Medical Institute, and the Sleep Disorders Center at Beth Israel Deaconess Medical Center—particularly Dr. Ann Webster, Dr. Margaret Caudill, Carol Wells-Federman, Eileen Stuart, and Dr. Jean Matheson—for sharing their ideas and talents, for their friendship and encouragement, and for helping to shape my thinking. Margaret Caudill suggested that I write this book, Jean Matheson provided me with the opportunity to join the Sleep Disorders Center at Beth Israel Deaconess Medical Center, and Ann Webster has brightened my days with her wisdom, energy, spirit, and encouragement.

The late Richard Friedman was my research director, mentor, colleague, and friend for ten years. His influence on my training and development as a scientist was immeasurable, as were his contributions to the field of behavioral medicine. His brilliance, spirit, and memory will live forever in my work and those of my colleagues at the Mind/Body Medical Institute.

I am also indebted to the many patients with whom I have worked over the past eighteen years. By sharing their experiences and lives with me, these individuals have helped me to grow as a clinician, scientist, and person. I also thank the administrative staff of the Division of Behavioral Medicine and the Sleep Disorders Center at the Beth Israel Deaconess Medical Center for their assistance with the Behavioral Medicine Insomnia Program; Joshua Sherman and George Warburg for their funding of my postdoctoral training; and the Paul P. Dosberg Foundation, Inc., and the National Institutes of Health for their research funding.

Thanks to Ned Leavitt and Connie Clausen for their suggestions in the preliminary phases of this project and to Deb Futter, Dr. Mitch Stein, Dr. Joan Borysenko, and Patti Breitman for their professional advice and assistance along the way.

Thanks also to my literary agent, Reid Boates. He believed in me and has made my first book an exciting, rewarding experience. His savvy advice, wisdom, and skill have been invaluable in every stage of this project. He is a delight to work with and the consummate professional.

A special thanks goes to my editor at Henry Holt, Tracy Brown, for his enthusiasm and confidence in me and for giving me the opportunity to write this book. Tracy's support and guidance made the somewhat daunting experience of writing my first book surprisingly painless. He is a writer's dream.

Finally, I am deeply grateful to my wife, Jody Skiest, and my father, Jim Jacobs, who encouraged me through every stage of this project, patiently reviewed every chapter of the manuscript, and offered invaluable feedback and suggestions on it. I could not have written this book without you.